Diabetes Management

Editor

LENNY SALZBERG

PRIMARY CARE: CLINICS IN OFFICE PRACTICE

www.primarycare.theclinics.com

Consulting Editor
JOEL J. HEIDELBAUGH

June 2022 • Volume 49 • Number 2

ELSEVIER

1600 John F. Kennedy Boulevard • Suite 1800 • Philadelphia, Pennsylvania, 19103-2899

http://www.theclinics.com

PRIMARY CARE: CLINICS IN OFFICE PRACTICE Volume 49, Number 2
June 2022 ISSN 0095-4543, ISBN-13: 978-0-323-84908-1

Editor: Katerina Heidhausen
Developmental Editor: Jessica Cañaberal

Primary Care: Clinics in Office Practice (ISSN: 0095-4543) is published quarterly by Elsevier Inc., 360 Park Avenue South, New York, NY 10010-1710. Months of issue are March, June, September, and December. Periodicals postage paid at New York, NY and additional mailing offices. Subscription prices are $269.00 per year (US individuals), $672.00 (US institutions), $100.00 (US students), $312.00 (Canadian individuals), $696.00 (Canadian institutions), $100.00 (Canadian students), $368.00 (international individuals), $696.00 (international institutions), and $175.00 (international students). Foreign air speed delivery is included in all *Clinics* subscription prices. All prices are subject to change without notice. POSTMASTER: Send address changes to *Primary Care: Clinics in Office Practice*, Elsevier Periodicals Customer Service, 11830 Westline Industrial Drive, St. Louis, MO 63146. Customer Service Health Sciences Division, Subscription Customer Service, 3251 Riverport Lane, Maryland Heights, MO 63043. **Customer Service: 1-800-654-2452 (U.S. and Canada); 314-447-8871 (outside U.S. and Canada). Fax: 314-447-8029. E-mail: journalscustomerservice-usa@elsevier.com (for print support); journalsonlinesupport-usa@elsevier.com (for online support).**

Reprints. For copies of 100 or more, of articles in this publication, please contact the Commercial Reprints Department, Elsevier Inc., 360 Park Avenue South, New York, NY 10010-1710. Tel. 212-633-3874; Fax: 212-633-3820; E-mail: reprints@elsevier.com.

Primary Care: Clinics in Office Practice is covered in *MEDLINE/PubMed (Index Medicus)* and *EMBASE/ Excerpta Medica, Current Contents/Clinical Medicine,* and *ISI/BIOMED.*

Contributors

CONSULTING EDITOR

JOEL J. HEIDELBAUGH, MD, FAAFP, FACG
Clinical Professor, Departments of Family Medicine and Urology, Director of Medical Student Education and Clerkship Director, Department of Family Medicine, University of Michigan Medical School, Ann Arbor, Michigan; Ypsilanti Health Center, Ypsilanti, Michigan

EDITOR

LENNY SALZBERG, MD, FAAFP
Diabetes Fellowship Director, Duke/Southern Regional Area Health Education Center, Fayetteville, North Carolina

AUTHORS

SUMERA AHMED, MD, BC-ADM
Assistant Professor, Primary Care Department, Program Director, Diabetes Fellowship, Touro University College of Osteopathic Medicine, Vallejo, California

DOYLE M. CUMMINGS, PharmD, FCP, FCCP
Department of Family Medicine, East Carolina University, Greenville, North Carolina

TAIWONA L. ELLIOTT, DO
Southern Regional Area Health Education Center, Fayetteville, North Carolina

AMBER M. HEALY, DO
Doctor of Osteopathic Medicine (DO), Assistant Clinical Professor, Diabetes Fellowship Program Director, Ohio University Heritage College of Osteopathic Medicine (OUHCOM), Ohio Health O'Bleness Memorial Hospital, Athens, Ohio

CECILIA C. LOW WANG, MD, FACP
Professor, Department of Medicine, Division of Endocrinology, Metabolism and Diabetes, Anschutz Medical Campus School of Medicine, Aurora, Colorado

MICHAEL MCRAE, DO
Family Medicine Physician and Diabetologist, St. Luke's Family Medicine, Nampa, Idaho

BASEM M. MISHRIKY, MD, FACP, ABOM
Diplomate, Diabetologist, Clinical Assistant Professor, Department of Internal Medicine, East Carolina University, Greenville, North Carolina

HEATHER O'BRIEN, PharmD, CPP
Clinical Pharmacy Faculty, Southern Regional Area Health Education Center, Fayetteville, North Carolina

SEAN M. OSER, MD, MPH
Associate Director, Practice Innovation Program of Colorado, Associate Director, Primary Care Diabetes Lab, Associate Professor, Department of Family Medicine, University of Colorado School of Medicine, Aurora, Colorado

TAMARA K. OSER, MD
Director, High Plains Research Network, Director, Primary Care Diabetes Lab, Associate Professor, Department of Family Medicine, University of Colorado School of Medicine, Aurora, Colorado

SHIVAJIRAO PRAKASH PATIL, MD, MPH, BC-ADM
Assistant Professor and Associate Director of Research, Department of Family Medicine, Brody School of Medicine, East Carolina University, Greenville, North Carolina

KIM M. PFOTENHAUER, DO, FACOFP
Assistant Professor, Michigan State University, College of Osteopathic Medicine, East Lansing, Michigan

BEATRIZ FRANCESCA RAMIREZ, MD
Medical Director of Inpatient Diabetes Management at Vidant Medical Center, Diabetes Fellowship Program Director, Clinical Assistant Professor of Endocrinology, Brody School of Medicine, East Carolina University, Greenville, North Carolina

STERLING RIDDLEY, MD
Fellowship Trained Diabetologist, Duke/Southern Regional Area Health Education Center, Fayetteville, North Carolina

LENNY SALZBERG, MD, FAAFP
Diabetes Fellowship Director, Duke/Southern Regional Area Health Education Center, Fayetteville, North Carolina

MICHAEL S. SHAPIRO, PhD
Director of Behavioral Medicine, Duke/Southern Regional Area Health Education Center, Fayetteville, North Carolina

JAY H. SHUBROOK, DO, FAAFP, FACOFP, BC-ADM
Professor, Primary Care Department, Touro University California, College of Osteopathic Medicine, Vallejo, California

KELSEY SIMMONS, DO
Fellowship Trained Diabetologist, Family Medicine, UNC Health Southeastern Gray's Creek Medical Clinic, Hope Mills, North Carolina

JOSEPH PATRICK STYERS, PharmD, BCPS, BCCCP
NorthBay Healthcare, Fairfield, California

JAMES R. POWELL, MD, FACP
Department of Internal Medicine, East Carolina University, Greenville, North Carolina

JULIA TECK, MD
Faculty Development Fellow, Duke/Southern Regional Area Health Education Center, Fayetteville, North Carolina

CATHERINE TRAVIS, PharmD, BCACP, CPP
Clinical Pharmacist, Cone Health, Greensboro, North Carolina

Contents

The incidence and prevalence of diabetes are increasing significantly globally and within the United States. Many individuals with diabetes are undiagnosed. The underlying causes of diabetes vary widely and are different in type 1 diabetes, type 2 diabetes, atypical diabetes, and gestational diabetes. It is important for clinicians to recognize the signs and symptoms of diabetes and use the proper diagnostic tools to diagnose diabetes.

There are many nonmodifiable and modifiable risk factors for type 2 diabetes. Nonmodifiable risk factors include age, genetics, epigenetics, and social determinants of health (including education level, socioeconomic status, and noise and arsenic exposure). Modifiable risk factors include obesity, the microbiome, diet, cigarette smoking, sleep duration, sleep quality, and sedentary behavior. Major lifestyle interventions to prevent and treat diabetes relate to these risk factors. Weight loss is the lifestyle intervention with the largest benefit for both preventing and treating diabetes. Exercise, even without weight loss, significantly reduces the incidence of type 2 diabetes.

Assessing glycemia over time remains a standard recommendation in the care of all people with diabetes. Glycemic assessment methods range from laboratory- and office-based methods to patient-based methods. Assessing A1c has long been the most common method of assessing overall glycemia. Continuous glucose monitoring (CGM) can also be used, especially via glucose management indicator or time-in-range, which can be useful especially when A1c might be impractical, unreliable, or inaccurate, or for glycemia assessment over a shorter interval. Other measures of glycemia, including hypoglycemia and glycemic variability, are becoming increasingly important in many cases and are also available via CGM.

> Type of diabetes is not always straightforward at presentation. Misdiagnosis is common in all age groups and diagnosis becomes evident over time. Patients with latent autoimmune diabetes in adults constitute up to 12% of all patients with diabetes, and they share immunogenetic and phenotypic features of type 1 and type 2 diabetes mellitus. They are commonly misdiagnosed as having type 2 diabetes mellitus, resulting in a delay in initiating insulin. Patients with ketosis-prone diabetes mellitus are often misdiagnosed as having type 1 diabetes mellitus. Correct diagnosis helps wean patients off of insulin and use noninsulin agents if needed.

> Diabetes-related microvascular complications include diabetic neuropathy (eg, diabetic symmetric polyneuropathy (DSPN), cardiac autonomic neuropathy, gastroparesis, enteropathy, erectile dysfunction, female sexual dysfunction, and hypoglycemia unawareness), diabetic kidney disease (DKD), and diabetes-related eye disease (eg, diabetic retinopathy (DR) and cataract). Both diabetes duration and degree of glycemic control strongly correlate with the development of microvascular complications. The development of diabetes-related microvascular complications interferes with the patient's quality of life and poses higher health system costs. This article will discuss a practical approach to effectively minimize/delay and manage the most common diabetes-related microvascular (DSPN, DKD, and DR).

> Because macrovascular complications of diabetes are the leading cause of mortality and decreased quality of life for individuals with diabetes, prevention and risk reduction are paramount. Besides lifestyle management, contemporary therapies can significantly reduce risk for cardiovascular events in diabetes. For primary prevention, most individuals should be on statin therapy, whereas those at high atherosclerotic cardiovascular disease risk should also be on glucagon-like peptide 1 receptor agonists (GLP1RA) or sodium/glucose cotransporter-2 inhibitors (SGLT2i) at any hemoglobin A1c. For secondary prevention, addition of GLP1RA or SGLT2i, PCKS9i, rivaroxaban, and/or icosapent ethyl should be considered in addition to a statin and low-dose aspirin.

> Diabetes influences other chronic medical conditions and is influenced by each in turn through multifactorial pathways. These comorbid conditions have a direct relationship with diabetes and can increase the severity of diabetes and the risk of various complications. Each of these comorbidities has unique recommendations for pharmaceutical treatment.

However, guidelines for all of these comorbidities also include lifestyle interventions as first-line treatment. Recent research has shown that diabetic medications may play a direct role in treating some of these comorbidities. This article focuses on the best-known comorbid diseases associated specifically with type 2 diabetes and their co-management.

PRIMARY CARE:
CLINICS IN OFFICE PRACTICE

SERIES OF RELATED INTEREST

Medical Clinics (http://www.medical.theclinics.com)
Physician Assistant Clinics (https://www.physicianassistant.theclinics.com)

THE CLINICS ARE AVAILABLE ONLINE!
Access your subscription at:
www.theclinics.com

Foreword

Comprehensive Diabetes Care

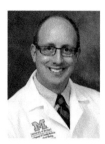

Joel J. Heidelbaugh, MD, FAAFP, FACG
Consulting Editor

In the era of panel management, I was surprised to learn that of nearly 2200 patients I provide primary care for, over 800 of these patients have diabetes. Many of these patients have complications of diabetes, and while many are well controlled, it is common for patients to inquire about new treatment and glucose-monitoring options. Certainly, the management of diabetes has changed dramatically since I finished training in the late 1990s. There are more oral medications, more insulins and insulin combinations, more novel classes of drugs, and avant-garde technology that allows for beaming your glucose reading to your cell phone and computer.

As Dr Salzberg highlights in his preface, the health care workforce is strained to meet the demand of endocrinologists to care for all of our diabetic patients. Moreover, primary care workforce shortages also abound despite the integration of more advanced practice providers. Clinical pharmacists are playing a large role in longitudinal management of our diabetic patients and helping to improve outcomes. This paradigm has expanded medical student and resident education to show a comprehensive and team-based approach to diabetes management.

I would like to thank Dr Salzberg and his authors for compiling a very complete guide to caring for diabetic patients in primary care practices and in the inpatient setting. Impressively, articles herein address both common and practical topics while expanding to more comprehensive subtopics across various populations. These include strategies for the care of pregnant women with diabetes, patients with disordered eating and depression, and those with common to more rare complications from diabetes. Sections on pharmacology highlight not only how medications work but also best indications and potential adverse effects. The article I learned the most from details resources for diabetic patients, which always seems to be a challenge, and the barriers are often moving targets. I hope that you will find this issue of *Primary Care: Clinics in*

Prim Care Clin Office Pract 49 (2022) xi–xii
https://doi.org/10.1016/j.pop.2021.12.005
0095-4543/22/© 2021 Published by Elsevier Inc.

Office Practice to be a useful and informative guide to comprehensive diabetes care with which to transform and augment the care of your diabetic patients.

Joel J. Heidelbaugh, MD, FAAFP, FACG
Departments of Family Medicine and Urology
University of Michigan Medical School
Ann Arbor, MI, USA

Ypsilanti Health Center
200 Arnet Suite 200
Ypsilanti, MI 48198, USA

E-mail address:
jheidel@umich.edu

Preface

Diabetes: A Growing Problem

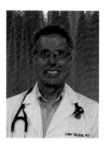

Lenny Salzberg, MD, FAAFP
Editor

As our country grows older and more obese, the number of people living with diabetes is increasing dramatically. While this is occurring, the pool of available endocrinologists and diabetologists (specialists trained to manage diabetes) has remained stable. Currently, roughly 85% of people with diabetes are treated by primary care physicians in primary care settings. This issue was written with you, the primary care provider, in mind.

The management of diabetes is complex. The purpose of this issue of *Primary Care: Clinics in Office Practice* is to help you understand this complexity to better care for your patients. The authors of these articles are a conglomeration of internists, family physicians, endocrinologists, pharmacists, and psychologists who were either trained in or teach in primary care diabetes fellowships. Our goal is to provide a clear, evidence-based, pragmatic roadmap for you to use to improve your patient care.

From prevention, to diagnosis, to treatment, we cover the bread-and-butter diabetes topics. Indications for using the different oral medications and the various injectable agents are clarified. How to choose the right insulin, and how to dose it in the office and in the hospital are described. We highlight the microvascular and macrovascular complications of diabetes, as well as diabetes-associated conditions, such as polycystic ovary syndrome and fatty liver. In addition to the basics, atypical diabetes (eg, LADA, MODY) diagnosis and management are reviewed, as are the implications and complications of diabetes in pregnancy. There is an article devoted to inpatient diabetes management, and one providing practical resources for patients (including links to on-line patient education resources and patient assistance programs). Psychosocial issues, including diabetes distress, depression, and disordered eating, are discussed. Rapidly changing technology, including insulin pumps, continuous glucose monitoring, and smart phone apps (among other advances) are addressed by two fellowship-trained diabetologists.

Prim Care Clin Office Pract 49 (2022) xiii–xiv
https://doi.org/10.1016/j.pop.2021.12.004
0095-4543/22/© 2021 Published by Elsevier Inc.

We hope this evidence-based, up-to-date issue helps you and your patients and increases your comfort with the ever-expanding specialty that is primary care diabetology.

This issue would not have been possible without the hard work and dedication of the authors. To them I am truly grateful. I would be remiss if I didn't give special recognition to Lisa Olsen Kilburn, MLIS, AHIP, SR-AHEC, Director of Library and Information Services, who did endless literature searches for the authors for five of these articles and was the first reader for many of the articles, mine included. Finally, I'd like to thank Grace Salzberg, who is currently a creative writing major at UNC-Asheville. Grace spent hours poring over the articles, helping improve our syntax, grammar, and flow.

Lenny Salzberg, MD, FAAFP
Duke Southern Regional Area
Health Education Center
1601 Owen Drive
Fayetteville, NC 28304, USA

E-mail address:
Lenny.Salzberg@sr-ahec.org

Classification and Diagnosis of Diabetes

Taiwona L. Elliott, DO[a],*, Kim M. Pfotenhauer, DO[b]

KEYWORDS

- Type 2 diabetes • Type 1 diabetes • Classification of diabetes
- Diagnosis of diabetes • Gestational diabetes • Atypical diabetes

KEY POINTS

- Type 1 diabetes is a result of an autoimmune T-cell–mediated attack on beta islet cells, resulting in insulin deficiency.
- There are multiple predisposing factors (eg, obesity, sedentary lifestyle, and high-risk ethnicities) that increase individuals' risk for prediabetes and type 2 diabetes development.
- Prediabetes, a precursor to diabetes, encompasses impaired glucose tolerance, elevated postprandial glucose levels, and impaired fasting glucose levels.
- Type 2 diabetes is defined as a progressive loss of beta-cell insulin secretion. It develops gradually over years and accounts for 90% to 95% of all diabetes. Type 2 diabetes has a myriad of effects on multiple organs.
- Four serum glucose tests are used to aid in diagnosing diabetes: fasting plasma glucose, 2-hour plasma glucose, 75 g oral glucose tolerance test, hemoglobin A1C, and random serum glucose.

INTRODUCTION

Diabetes is estimated to affect approximately 34.2 million individuals in the United States. Approximately 21.4% of these, or 7.3 million people, are undiagnosed.[1] Diabetes presents across multiple clinical settings (eg, emergency departments, urgent care facilities, and outpatient clinics) with a multiple different clinical presentations and symptoms. Classification should be determined so effective treatment can be implemented.

---

[a] Southern Regional Area Health Education Center, 1601 Owen Dr., Fayetteville, NC 28303, USA; [b] Michigan State University, College of Osteopathic Medicine, Rm 325, 965 Wilson Rd, East Lansing, MI 48824, USA
* Corresponding author.
E-mail address: Taiwona.elliott@sr-ahec.org

Prim Care Clin Office Pract 49 (2022) 191–200
https://doi.org/10.1016/j.pop.2021.11.011
primarycare.theclinics.com

Classification

Diabetes is classified into 4 groups by the American Diabetes Association: type 1, type 2, specific types of diabetes due to other causes (sometimes called atypical diabetes), and gestational diabetes[2] (**Table 1**).

TYPE 1 DIABETES
Epidemiology

Type 1 diabetes accounts for 5% to 10% of diabetes cases with an increasing incidence and a global prevalence of 2% annually.[3,4] In the United States, the incidence is 20 cases per 100,000 people among those younger than 65 years.[4] Many of the mutations causing type 1 diabetes are inherited; the disease concordance in identical twins is 30% to 70%.[3] Environmental or behavioral factors, such as the infant and adult diet, decreased gut-microbiome heterogeneity, and early exposure to viruses associated with islet cell inflammation[4] are thought to be the cause for the increasing incidence of type 1 diabetes.

Pathophysiology

Type 1 diabetes is defined as "autoimmune beta-cell destruction usually leading to absolute insulin deficiency."[2] This form of diabetes has traditionally been thought of as presenting in children and was previously called juvenile diabetes. Although most of the patients still present around this age, there is also a second spike of diagnoses in adults aged 35 to 50 years. This presentation in adults is called latent autoimmune diabetes of the adult (LADA).

Type 1 diabetes results from a T-cell–mediated attack on pancreatic islet beta cells. The classic presentation of diabetic ketoacidosis usually occurs when 90% of beta cells are not functioning. The disease has strong human leukocyte antigen associations and numerous antibody markers. Type 1 diabetes is further classified into 3 distinct stages. The autoimmune markers vary, but when more than 2 are present and the person is normoglycemic, an individual is considered as having stage 1.[2] Stage 2 presents with autoantibodies and dysglycemia, but this stage is often missed as the individual is still asymptomatic.[2] Stage 3 occurs with new-onset hyperglycemia, clinical symptoms, and autoantibodies present[2] (**Table 2**). Frequently, type 1 diabetes is diagnosed during stage 3, when individuals are noted to have classic hyperglycemic systems (polyuria, polydipsia, and weight loss); approximately one-third of patients present with diabetic ketoacidosis.[3]

Table 1	
Diabetes types and causes	
Type of Diabetes	**Cause**
Type 1 diabetes	Autoimmune β-cell destruction, usually leading to absolute insulin deficiency
Type 2 diabetes	Progressive loss of adequate β-cell insulin secretion frequently on the background of insulin resistance
Diabetes due to other causes	Monogenic diabetes, diseases of the exocrine pancreas, drug- or chemical-induced diabetes
Gestational diabetes	Diabetes diagnosed in the second or third trimester of pregnancy that was not overt diabetes before gestation.

Data from American Diabetes Association Diabetes Care 2021 Jan; 44(Supplement 1): S15-S33. Available at: https://care.diabetesjournals.org/content/44/Supplement_1/S15.article-info.

Table 2 Stages of type 1 diabetes			
Stage	**Autoantibody Detected**	**Serum Blood Glucose Levels**	**Symptoms**
Stage 1	≥2 autoantibodies present	Normoglycemia	Asymptomatic
Stage 2	≥2 autoantibodies present	Dysglycemic	Asymptomatic
Stage 3	≥2 autoantibodies present	Hyperglycemic	Symptomatic

Data from American Diabetes Association Diabetes Care 2021 Jan; 44(Supplement 1): S15-S33. Available at: https://care.diabetesjournals.org/content/44/Supplement_1/S15.article-info.

Type 1 diabetes is further divided into type 1A and 1B. Type 1A presents with the classic signs and symptoms of insulin deficiency with either glutamic acid decarboxylase antibodies or islet cell antibodies present. Type 1B also begins with the classic presentation but typical antibody markers are not present. However, zinc transporter antibodies are present in type 1B.[5] Those with LADA typically present with a slower beta-cell loss and are often misdiagnosed with type 2 diabetes.

Prediabetes

An estimated 88 million Americans have prediabetes with only 15.3% diagnosed.[1] Typically, impaired glucose tolerance is the first dysfunction seen on the continuum of type 2 diabetes. Before hyperglycemia is seen in the fasting glucose, an increase in the postprandial glucose occurs. Prediabetes is a term used to identify individuals whose glucose levels do not meet the criteria for diabetes diagnosis but are greater than the normal ranges.[6] Individuals with prediabetes have an increased risk of developing type 2 diabetes and cardiovascular disease. Macrovascular and microvascular changes are commonly seen at diagnosis of type 2 diabetes because of the gradual onset of the disease that often goes unrecognized.[2] Prediabetes should not be viewed as its own clinical entity, but as a precursor to diabetes development.[1]

Prediabetes is defined by multiple criteria: impaired glucose tolerance (140–199 mg/dL), impaired fasting glucose (100–125 mg/dL), or abnormal hemoglobin A1C (5.7%–6.4%).[7] (**Table 3**). Only one abnormal finding for the 3 outlined criteria is needed to diagnose prediabetes. Progression to diabetes is disproportionately greater at the higher end of the abnormal ranges.[2] A systematic review of 16 cohort studies found individuals with higher A1C values (6.0%–6.5%) had substantially increased risk of diabetes development at 5 years (25%–50%), demonstrating the importance of screening and early detection.[8]

Table 3 Criteria for prediabetes (1 of the 3 needed)	
Criteria For Prediabetes (1 of the 3 needed)	
Fasting Plasma Glucose	100 mg/dL to 125 mg/dL
75 gram oral glucose tolerance test (OGTT)	140 mg/dL to 199 mg/dL
Hemoglobin A1C	5.7% to 6.4%

Data from American Diabetes Association Diabetes Care 2021 Jan; 44(Supplement 1): S15-S33. Available at: https://care.diabetesjournals.org/content/44/Supplement_1/S15.article-info.

TYPE 2 DIABETES

Type 2 diabetes is defined as a progressive loss of beta-cell insulin secretion on the background of insulin resistance; this develops gradually over years and accounts for 90% to 95% of all diabetes.[2] Typically thought of as adult-onset diabetes, prediabetes and type 2 diabetes are now also becoming more common in young adults and youth.

In addition to hyperglycemia and insulin resistance, type 2 diabetes causes several other metabolic effects. Alpha cells of the pancreas show resistance to insulin so they do not inhibit glucagon release during meals. There is accelerated lipolysis in adipocytes, increased glucose reabsorption in the kidneys, increased hepatic glucose production, and decreased incretin effects. In addition, neural dysregulation in the brain leads to increased appetite, decreased morning dopamine surge, and increased sympathetic tone.[9]

Postprandial glucose is regulated by the food bolus, timing of insulin release, and glucose suppression. Hepatic, adipose, and muscle tissue respond to insulin by increasing the uptake of glucose and suppressing gluconeogenesis. In type 2 diabetes, insulin resistance impairs this response, leading to postprandial hyperglycemia. Hepatic glucose production (gluconeogenesis) is a primary factor in determining fasting plasma glucose. Gluconeogenesis is regulated by fasting plasma insulin, hepatic sensitivity to insulin, fasting substrate availability, and glucagon levels. In type 2 diabetes, elevated fasting glucose results from basal insulin secretion impairment, decreased hepatic sensitivity to insulin, increased circulating lipids, and increased glucagon levels.[9]

DIAGNOSIS OF DIABETES
Diagnostic and Screening Criteria for Diabetes

There are multiple risks increasing the development of prediabetes and type 2 diabetes, with overweight, obesity, and sedentary lifestyle confirmed as environmental risk factors and ethnicity and family history noted as genetic factors.[10] **Box 1** outlines screening criteria for diabetes and prediabetes in asymptomatic adults. The American Diabetes Association has developed an online risk-assessment tool (diabetes.org/socrisktest) to aid with performing diagnostic testing.[2]

Type 2 Diabetes Diagnosis

Four serum glucose tests are used to aid in diagnosing diabetes: fasting plasma glucose, 2-hour plasma glucose (2-h PG) 75 g oral glucose tolerance test (OGTT), hemoglobin A1C (HbA1C), and random serum glucose with classic symptom of polyuria, polydipsia, or hyperglycemic crisis (**Table 4**). The diagnosis of diabetes should be confirmed with a repeat abnormal test using the same blood sample or another sample using any of the serum glucose testing methods.[11] If a second sample is used, the test should be completed expeditiously to confirm the diagnosis and the diagnosis made based on the confirmatory test.[2] Patients with classic symptoms of diabetes (polydipsia, polyuria, and polyphagia) or hyperglycemic crisis and a random blood glucose greater than or equal to 200 mg/dL do not require confirmatory testing.[2]

The 2-h PG test should be performed in accordance with the World Health Organization's guidelines, using a glucose load containing 75 g of anhydrous glucose dissolved in water. This test is infrequently used by primary care clinicians due to the time requirements, but the 2-h PG is more sensitive for diagnoses of prediabetes and diabetes compared with HbA1C.[12] HbA1C has become the favored test for many primary care clinicians, as the test does not require fasting or timed samples

---

Box 1
Screening criteria for diabetes and prediabetes in asymptomatic adults

1. Universal screening at 45 years; if normal, repeat at 3-y intervals

2. Risk factor–based testing for overweight or obesity (BMI $\geq$25 kg/m^3 or $\geq$ 23 kg/m^3 in Asian Americans) in individuals with one or more risk factors:
   a. Sedentary lifestyle
   b. First-degree relative with diabetes
   c. High-risk ethnicity/race (eg, African American, Latino, Hispanic American, Native American, Asian American, Pacific Islander)
   d. Hypertension (blood pressure $\geq$140/90 mm Hg or on antihypertensive medication)
   e. HDL $\leq$35 mg/dL (0.9 mmol/L)
   f. Triglycerides $\geq$259 mg/dL (2.82 mmol/L)
   g. Clinic conditions associated with insulin resistance (eg, PCOS, acanthosis nigrans [60%–90% in T2DM])

3. History of GDM: lifelong testing every 3 y

4. Diagnosis of HIV: annual screening

5. Annual testing for prediabetes

Abbreviations: BMI, body mass index; GDM, gestational diabetes mellitus; HDL, high-density lipoprotein; HIV, human immunodeficiency virus; PCOS, polycystic ovary syndrome; T2DM, type 2 diabetes mellitus.

Adapted from American Diabetes Association Diabetes Care 2021 Jan; 44(Supplement 1): S15-S33. Available at: https://care.diabetesjournals.org/content/44/Supplement_1/S15.article-info.

---

and has a better overall glycemic exposure assessment, but the test has a low sensitivity for identifying diabetes and prediabetes compared with the 2-h PG and fasting plasma glucose test.[12]

HbA1C is an indirect measure of average blood glucose levels, and multiple factors can affect hemoglobin glycation independent of hyperglycemia[2] (**Box 2**). Conditions with increased red blood cell turnover or loss, such as sickle cell anemia, pregnancy, hemodialysis, recent blood loss, or transfusion, result in less reliable HbA1C measurements.[13] Studies show HbA1C levels are affected by protease inhibitors (PI) and nucleoside reverse transcriptase inhibitors (NNRTI) in human immunodeficiency virus (HIV) individuals, but the ease and specificity of the test warrant continued use in patients with HIV treated with PI and NNRTI.[14]

Table 4
Diagnostic for diabetes mellitus (requires only 1 positive value)

Plasma Glucose	Diabetes Mellitus
Fasting[a]	$\geq$ 126 mg/dL (7.0 mmol/L)
2-h 75g OGTT	$\geq$200 mg/dL (11.1 mmol/L)
HbA1C	$\geq$6.5% (48 mmol/mol)
Random[b] plus polydipsia, polyphagia, polyuria, or hyperglycemic crisis	$\geq$200 mg/dL (11.1 mmol/L)

[a] Fasting defined as no solid or liquid food, except water, for at least 8 h.
[b] Random refers to any time of day, unrelated to meals.
Data from American Diabetes Association Diabetes Care 2021 Jan; 44(Supplement 1): S15-S33. Available at: https://care.diabetesjournals.org/content/44/Supplement_1/S15.article-info.

| Box 2 |
Factors affecting hemoglobin glycation
Hemodialysis
Pregnancy
HIV (treated with antiretrovirals): PI therapy increased HbA1C levels
NNRTI therapy decreased HbA1C levels
Iron-deficient anemia
Hemoglobinopathies (HbS, G6PD): decrease HbA1C by 0.3%–0.8%
Erythropoietin therapy
Data from Refs.[2,12]

ATYPICAL DIABETES

Atypical diabetes is a group of diseases that can be attributed to specific causes. This group includes monogenic diabetes, diseases of the exocrine pancreas, and drug- or chemical-induced diabetes. Taken together, these forms make up a small percentage of those diagnosed with diabetes.

Monogenic diabetes is a form of diabetes that results from beta-cell defects due to gene mutations. Mutations in these genes result in impaired glucose sensing or impaired insulin secretion with minimal or no defect in insulin action. Because this group of diabetes is genetic, it is usually diagnosed in younger populations. Neonatal diabetes usually presents in those younger than 6 months, and monogenic diabetes of the young (MODY) usually presents in those younger than 25 years.[2]

Neonatal diabetes can be either transient or permanent. Transient forms are most often due to an overexpression of genes on chromosome 6q24; this type can recur in about half of the cases. Permanent forms are most commonly due to autosomal dominant mutations of beta-cell K-ATP channels. Mutations on the gene that codes insulin itself is the second most common cause.[2]

MODY is an autosomal dominant disease that is characterized by noninsulin-dependent diabetes diagnosed at a young age (younger than 25 years). The most common form, MODY 3, is due to an HNF-1α defect. Clinically, high postprandial blood glucose is most commonly seen. Treatment is with sulfonylureas, not insulin. MODY 2, caused by a defect in glucokinase, is the second most common form. Clinically, mild, stable fasting hyperglycemia is most commonly seen and can be misdiagnosed as prediabetes or type 2 diabetes on routine screening. Unlike type 2 diabetes, this form of diabetes is not progressive.[2]

Diseases of the exocrine pancreas include diabetes due to cystic fibrosis (CF), pancreatitis (acute and chronic), trauma or pancreatectomy, neoplasia, or hemochromatosis. Diabetes is the most common comorbidity of cystic fibrosis, occurring in 40% to 50% of adults with CF. Clinically, patients present with insulin insufficiency, insulin resistance, and impaired glucose tolerance. Drug- or chemical-induced diabetes can be caused due to posttransplantation immunosuppressive therapies, HIV antiretrovirals, or glucocorticoids.[2]

GESTATIONAL DIABETES

Diabetes is one of the most common medical complications of pregnancy; this can be due to preexisting type 1 or type 2 diabetes or diabetes that develops during pregnancy. The incidence of diabetes complicating pregnancy has increased about 40% in the last 20 years. Gestational diabetes is defined as diabetes that is diagnosed in the second or third trimester of pregnancy that was not clearly overt diabetes before pregnancy.[2] Currently, approximately 7% of pregnancies are complicated by diabetes, 90% of which are classified as gestational diabetes.[15] It is important to screen and diagnose diabetes in pregnancy due to the many maternal and fetal complications (**Table 5**).

In early pregnancy, higher levels of estrogen enhance insulin sensitivity, often resulting in hypoglycemia. By the second and third trimesters, increasing hyperglycemia can be seen due to insulin resistance mediated by placental hormones such as placental growth hormone, cortisol, human placental lactogen, progesterone, and prolactin.[15]

Diagnosis and treatment of gestational diabetes are important to reduce the consequences for both the infant and the mother (see **Table 5**). Infants can develop macrosomia that can lead to traumatic deliveries including shoulder dystocia, brachial plexus injuries, or clavicular factures. Delayed organ maturity, organomegaly, and polycythemia can also be complications. Because glucose can cross the placenta but maternal insulin cannot, infants can overproduce insulin after birth, leading to hypoglycemia, electrolyte disturbances, jittery and irritable neonates, poor feeding, or seizures. Long-term, infants born to mothers with gestational diabetes are at a higher risk for obesity, diabetes, impaired fine and gross motor function, and increased rates of attention deficit hyperactivity disorder. There can also be maternal consequences of gestational diabetes including higher rates of polyhydramnios, preeclampsia, complications of traumatic delivery, and higher rates of cesarean sections. Mothers with gestational diabetes can also experience complications typically seen in other forms of diabetes including hypoglycemia, worsening end-organ damage, infections, or ketoacidosis.[15]

Table 5	
Maternal and infant consequences of gestational diabetes	
Maternal Consequences	Infant Consequences
Polyhydramnios	Macrosomia
Preeclampsia	Traumatic delivery
Traumatic delivery	Shoulder dystocia
Operative delivery	Brachial plexus injuries
Hypoglycemia	Clavicular factures
End-organ damage	Delayed organ maturity
Increased infections	Organomegaly
Ketoacidosis	Polycythemia
Increased risk of developing T2DM	Hypoglycemia after birth
—	Electrolyte disturbances
—	Jittery, irritability
—	Poor feeding
—	Seizures

Data from Practice Bulletin No. 180: Gestational Diabetes Mellitus. Obstet Gynecol. 2017 Jul;130(1):e17-e37.

Diagnosing Gestational Diabetes

All pregnant patients should be screened for gestational diabetes at 24 to 28 weeks gestation. The American College of Obstetricians and Gynecologists recommends screening for diabetes at the first prenatal visit in patients with a body mass index greater than or equal to 25 kg/m^3 and one type 2 diabetes risk factor using the testing methods outlined in **Table 4** (eg, fasting blood glucose, 2-H 75g OGTT, or HbA1C).[15] Patients with normal early prenatal screening should undergo repeat screening at 24 to 28 weeks using the one-step or two-step method.

TESTING METHODS
Two-Step Method

The two-step method recommended by the National Institutes of Health and commonly used in the United States requires a 1-hour nonfasting 50-g glucose loading test followed by a 3-hour fasting 100-g OGTT for patients with a positive 1-hour 50-g test. The thresholds for the 1-hour glucose challenge test vary from 130 mg/dL, 135 mg/dL, to 140 mg/dL. The variation in positive thresholds for the 1-hour 50-g test is due to a lack of randomized trials examining if one cutoff shows improved pregnancy outcomes. Frequently, the 140 mg/dL cutoff is used due to high specificity, 69% to 89%, and lower rates of false-positive screening results compared with the 130 mg/dL cutoff (66%–77% specific).[2,15]

Patients with a positive 1-hour test should undergo a 3-hour diagnostic OGTT. The OGTT requires patients to fast and is considered positive for gestational diabetes if 2 values are abnormal. Two different criteria, the National Diabetes Data Group and Carpenter and Coustan (**Table 6**), are used to interpret the 3-hour OGTT. The Carpenter-Coustan threshold values are lower and result in higher rates of gestational diabetes diagnoses. There are no clear comparative studies demonstrating the superiority of the 2 diagnostic criteria.[15]

One-Step Method

The one-step method is recommended by the International Association of Diabetes and Pregnancy Study Group. The approach requires a 75-g 2-hour OGTT with a single

Table 6
Criteria for gestational diabetes mellitus

Status	Plasma or Serum Glucose Level Carpenter and Coustan Conversion		Plasma Level National Diabetes Data Group Conversion	
	mg/dL	mmol/L	mg/dL	mmol/L
Fasting	95	5.3	105	5.8
1 h	180	10.0	190	10.6
2 h	155	8.6	165	9.2
3 h	140	7.8	145	8.0

A diagnosis generally requires that 2 or more thresholds be met or exceeded, although some clinicians choose to use just 1 elevated value.

Adapted from the American Diabetes Association. Classification and Diagnosis of Diabetes. Diabetes Care 2017;40 (Suppl. 1):S11-S24.Copyright 2017 American Diabetes Association.*From* Practice Bulletin No. 180: Gestational Diabetes Mellitus. Obstet Gynecol. 2017 Jul;130(1):e17-e37; with permission.

Table 7 One-step: 75-g 2-hour oral glucose tolerance test	
Status	Serum Glucose Level
Fasting	≥ 92 mg/dL
1 h	≥ 180 mg/dL
2 h	≥ 153 mg/dL
Gestational diabetes diagnosed with one positive value	

Data from Practice Bulletin No. 180: Gestational Diabetes Mellitus. Obstet Gynecol. 2017 Jul;130(1):e17-e37.

positive value at fasting greater than or equal to 92 mg/dL, 1-h greater than or equal to 180 mg/dL, or 2-h greater than or equal to 153 mg/dL (**Table 7**). The one-step approach results in higher gestational diabetes diagnosis rates with no clear evidence supporting improved maternal or neonatal outcomes and may result in increased health care costs.[15]

CLINICS CARE POINTS

- If a patient has increased red blood cell turnover or loss, consider screening for prediabetes or diabetes with the OGTT, a fasting glucose, or a random glucose. Hemoglobin A1C measurements are less reliable in this patient subset.
- If a patient has screened positive for diabetes, a confirmatory test should be done expeditiously using any of the testing methods: fasting serum glucose, oral glucose tolerance test, hemoglobin A1C, or a random glucose.
- Pregnant patients screened at their initial visit for diabetes should undergo repeat screening at 24 to 28 weeks using either the one-step or the two-step method.

DISCLOSURE

Neither author has a commercial or financial conflict of interest.

REFERENCES

1. Centers for Disease Control and Prevention. National diabetes Statistics, 2020: Estimates of diabetes and its burden in the United States. Atlanta, (GA): Centers for Disease Control and Prevention, United States Department of Health and Human Services; 2020. Accessed July 15 2021.
2. American diabetes association Standards of medical care in diabetes. Available at: https://care.diabetesjournals.org/content/44/supplement_1. Accessed July 15 2021.
3. DiMeglio LA, Evans-Molina C, Oram RA. Type 1 diabetes. Lancet 2018; 391(10138):2449–62.
4. Mobasseri M, Shirmohammadi M, Amiri T, et al. Prevalence and incidence of type 1 diabetes in the world: a systematic review and meta-analysis. Health Promot Perspect 2020;10(2):98–115.
5. Paschou SA, Papadopoulou-Marketou N, Chrousos GP, et al. On type 1 diabetes mellitus pathogenesis. Endocr Connect 2018;7(1):R38–46.

6. Selvin E, Rawlings AM, Bergenstal RM, et al. No racial differences in the association of glycated hemoglobin with kidney disease and cardiovascular outcomes. Diabetes Care 2013;36:2995–3001.

7. Expert Committee on the Diagnosis and Classification of Diabetes Mellitus. Report of the Expert Committee on the Diagnosis and Classification of Diabetes Mellitus. Diabetes Care 1997;20:1183–97.

8. Zhang X, Gregg EW, Williamson DF, et al. A1C level and future risk of diabetes: a systematic review. Diabetes Care 2010;33(7):1665–73.

9. Defronzo RA. Banting Lecture: From the triumvirate to the ominous octet: a new paradigm for the treatment of type 2 diabetes mellitus. Diabetes 2009;58:773–95.

10. Khan RMM, Chua ZJY, Tan JC, et al. From Pre-Diabetes to Diabetes: Diagnosis, Treatments and Translational Research. Medicina 2019;55(9):546. https://doi.org/10.3390/medicina55090546.

11. Selvin E, Wang D, Matsushita K, et al. Prognostic Implications of Single-Sample Confirmatory Testing for Undiagnosed Diabetes: A Prospective Cohort Study. Ann Intern Med 2018;169(3):156–64.

12. Meijnikman AS, De Block CEM, Dirinck E, et al. Not performing an OGTT results in significant underdiagnosis of (pre)diabetes in a high risk adult Caucasian population. Int J Obes (Lond) 2017;41(11):1615–20.

13. Guo F, Moellering DR, Garvey WT. Use of HbA1c for diagnoses of diabetes and prediabetes: comparison with diagnoses based on fasting and 2-hr glucose values and effects of gender, race, and age. Metab Syndr Relat Disord 2014;12(5):258–68.

14. Eckhardt BJ, Holzman RS, Kwan CK, et al. Glycated Hemoglobin A(1c) as screening for diabetes mellitus in HIV-infected individuals. AIDS Patient Care STDS 2012;26(4):197–201.

15. Practice Bulletin No. 180: Gestational Diabetes Mellitus. Obstetrics & Gynecology 2017;130(1):e17–37.

Risk Factors and Lifestyle Interventions

Lenny Salzberg, MD, FAAFP

KEYWORDS

- Risk factors • Lifestyle interventions • Diets • Diabetes prevention program

KEY POINTS

- Age, genetics, epigenetics, and social determinants of health are significant risk factors for diabetes
- Obesity, the gut microbiome, diet, cigarette smoking, sleep (duration and quality), and sedentary behavior are modifiable risk factors for diabetes
- The lifestyle intervention with the largest benefit for both preventing and treating diabetes is weight loss
- Exercise, even without weight loss, reduces the incidence of type 2 diabetes

The prevalence of diabetes is increasing rapidly, doubling between 1980 and 2014 (adjusted for the impact of aging),[1] paralleling the obesity epidemic. Understanding the risk factors for diabetes dovetails with choosing appropriate lifestyle interventions for both prevention and treatment. The primary focus of this article will be on risk factors and lifestyle interventions for patients with type 2 diabetes.

RISK FACTORS

Age

Age is a significant risk factor for type 2 diabetes. Worldwide, the number of adults with diabetes quadrupled between 1980 and 2014, from 108 million to 422 million,[1] with half of this increase due to the aging of the population. More than 50% of older adults have prediabetes, and more than a quarter of people in the United States ≥ 65 years of age have type 2 diabetes.[2] Aging is inevitable and not modifiable.

Obesity

The most important modifiable risk factor for diabetes is obesity. Some describe the global explosion of diabetes incidence as the "Diabesity Epidemic."[3] There is a 50- to 80-fold increased relative risk for type 2 diabetes in men with a BMI over 35 kg/m2 compared with men with a BMI of less than 23 kg/m2 (in populations of white European descent).[4] Obesity does not necessarily cause diabetes, but it is correlated.

Duke/ Southern Regional Area Health Education Center, 1601 Owen Drive, Fayetteville, NC 28304, USA
E-mail address: Lenny.Salzberg@sr-ahec.org

Prim Care Clin Office Pract 49 (2022) 201–212
https://doi.org/10.1016/j.pop.2021.11.001
0095-4543/22/© 2021 Elsevier Inc. All rights reserved.

This correlation of obesity and diabetes, however, is not 1:1; there are "healthy" obese patients and unhealthy normal weight or overweight patients. The location of fat may be more important than the total amount of fat; ectopic fat seems to drive type 2 diabetes. Ectopic fat, defined as the storage of triglycerides in tissues that normally store only small amounts of fat, has been best studied in the liver but also occurs in the heart, in skeletal muscle, and in the pancreas.[5] Pancreatic fat may cause beta-cell dysfunction,[6] leading to diabetes. Support for the ectopic fat hypothesis comes from patients with lipodystrophy who have an impaired ability to store fat in the subcutaneous space. When these patients have even modest weight gain, they accumulate fat in visceral tissues, leading to marked insulin resistance[7] and eventually diabetes. Epidemiologic studies show that, as compared with women at most ages, men develop diabetes at lower average BMI and have more liver (ectopic) fat than women at comparable BMI. In addition, South Asians develop type 2 diabetes at lower BMI levels (and a decade earlier in life) than white Europeans,[8] and they also have proportionately more ectopic fat.

Genetics

Genetics is our DNA sequence. Genome-wide association (GWA) scans have helped identify 500 gene loci associated with susceptibility for type 2 diabetes. These genes predominantly affect pancreatic beta-cell development and function, and to a lesser extent obesity and insulin resistance. Together, these genes account for 20% of the predisposition to type 2 diabetes.[9] Obesity, and therefore diabetes, is related to energy balance (energy intake through energy-dense diets[10] and energy output via physical (in) activity), and also to genetic factors, epigenetic factors, and the gut microbiome.

Epigenetics

Epigenetics is the genomic control mechanism resulting from changes in the structure of chromatin (the macromolecules found in the cell nucleus) without changes to the DNA sequence.[11] These stable and heritable changes are caused by DNA methylation, small interfering RNAs, and histone (protein) posttranslational modifications. Epigenetics is influenced by aging, the environment, and exposures *in utero*.[12]

The relationship between prenatal exposures and diabetes risk has led to the formulation of the Developmental Origins of Health and Disease (DOHaD) hypothesis.[13] Prenatal exposure to famine is associated with a higher risk of developing type 2 diabetes.[14] Low birth weight has the same association.[15] Animal studies show various models of intrauterine growth restriction (IUGR) cause profound changes in pancreas, liver, skeletal muscle and adipose tissue, associated with abnormal glucose metabolism.[13] Animal models and epidemiologic studies show the same for maternal gestational diabetes and maternal obesity leading to diabetes in offspring.[13] In women with gestational diabetes, there is a 7- to 8-fold higher risk of their children developing diabetes, associated with several epigenetic modifications.

Transgenerational epigenetics (the transfer of epigenetic marks from one generation to another), independent of that individual's in utero conditions, occurs and also might be contributing to the logarithmic growth of the diabetes epidemic.

Microbiome

One of the frontiers in diabetes risk stratification is the complex gut ecosystem, which maintains a symbiotic relationship with the gut mucosa. Gut bacteria are involved in nutrient metabolism, drug metabolism, maintenance of structural integrity of the gut mucosal barrier, immunomodulation, and protection against pathogens. Dysbiosis, an imbalance in gut microbiota, occurs when there is an unhealthy diet, antibiotic treatment, or chronic infection. Eating an animal-based diet rapidly and reproducibly decreases the abundance of Firmicutes, one of the key bacteria in the gut microbiome.[16] Animal-based diets (compared with plant-based diets) are associated with diabetes.

Dietary carbohydrates are fermented in the colon by gut bacteria, giving rise to butyrate and other short-chain fatty acids (SCFAs). SCFAs can account for up to 10% of a person's total caloric intake per day[17] while also acting as signaling molecules that affect metabolism, energy balance, and immune homeostasis. The gut microbiome in patients with prediabetes and diabetes is different from that of normal controls, with decreased levels of butyrate-producing bacteria.[17] Strategies to prevent and treat diabetes through the manipulation of the gut microbiota are being developed.

Diabetes-protective Diets

Despite a plethora of studies, there are many questions about the best diet to prevent and treat prediabetes and diabetes. In the 2021 Diabetes Standards of Medical Care, the American Diabetes Association concluded that "…there is not an ideal percentage of calories from carbohydrate, protein, and fat for all people to prevent diabetes; therefore, macronutrient distribution should be based on an individualized assessment of current eating patterns, preferences and metabolic goals."[18] Weight loss and reduced total calorie intake lead to better glycemic control[19]; as do specific eating patterns without weight loss.

Specific eating patterns that lead to better glycemic control (hemoglobin A1c reduction of 0.12%–0.5% compared with comparison or control diets) include the Mediterranean diet, low-carbohydrate diets, low glycemic index (GI) diets, and high-protein diets; with the largest effect size seen in the Mediterranean diet.[19]

In the landmark PREDIMED-Reus nutrition intervention trial, 418 nondiabetic subjects aged 55 to 80 were randomized to a traditional Mediterranean diet with the liberal addition of virgin olive oil, a traditional Mediterranean diet with mixed nuts (30 g per day) added daily, or a control group on a low-fat diet. After a 4-year follow-up, diabetes incidence was 10.1% in the olive oil group, 11.0% in the nuts group, and 17.9% in the control group. When the Mediterranean diet groups were pooled, diabetes incidence was reduced by 52% compared with the control group. Interestingly, diabetes risk reduction occurred in the absence of significant changes in body weight or physical activity. In the study, behavioral interventions promoting the Mediterranean diet were implemented and personalized dietary advice was given to participants (**Box 1**).[20]

In the PREDIMED trial, people who were alcohol drinkers were encouraged to continue moderate consumption of red wine, defined as 1 to 2 drinks per day in women and 2 to 3 drinks per day in men, as part of the Mediterranean diet. In a review article, Golan, and colleagues describe that the metabolic syndrome is significantly more common in nondrinkers than among wine drinkers, and conclude that initiating moderate alcohol consumption is safe in patients with well-controlled type 2 diabetes.[21]

In addition to the diets mentioned above, the Dietary Approaches to Stop Hypertension (DASH) eating patterns,[22] vegetarian diets,[23] and plant-based diets[24] are associated with a lower risk of developing type 2 diabetes. The quality of food consumed, as measured by the Healthy Eating Index (HEI), the Alternative Healthy Eating Index (AHEI), and the DASH score, is also associated with a lower risk of type 2 diabetes[25] (**Box 2**).

Box 1
Dietary advice for the Mediterranean diet

1) Abundant use of virgin olive oil for cooking and dressing (1 L per week was provided to study participants)

2) Increased consumption of fruit, vegetables, legumes, and fish

3) Reduction in total meat consumption, less processed meat, less red meat

4) Preparation of homemade sauce with tomato, garlic, onion, and spices with olive oil

5) Avoidance of butter, cream, fast food, sweets, pastries, and sugar-sweetened beverages

6) In alcohol drinkers, moderate consumption of red wine

After water, coffee is the second most consumed beverage world-wide. Both caffeinated and decaffeinated coffee intake has an inverse relationship with diabetes incidence: the more coffee consumed, the less likely you are to become diabetic. There are many proposed mechanisms for this, including effects on enzymes that metabolize insulin and glucose. The Pan-American Health Organization and the American Regional Office of the World Health Organization (WHO) recommend that we drink 3 to 4 cups of coffee per day![26]

Cinnamon has been studied extensively as a dietary supplement for use as a complementary treatment of diabetes.[27] When added to conventional medication and lifestyle changes, cinnamon has only modest effects on fasting glucose and on hemoglobin A1c. The National Institutes of Health (NIH) National Center for Complementary and Integrative Health does not recognize the use of cinnamon for either treatment or prevention of diabetes.[28]

Cigarette Smoking

Cigarette smoking is bad for you. Smoking causes cancer, pulmonary disease (COPD), and cardiovascular disease. Per *The Health Consequences of Smoking – 50 Years of*

Box 2
Components of quality food

Healthy Eating Index (HEI-2015)	Alternative Healthy Eating Index (A-HEI)	Dietary Approaches to Stop Hypertension (DASH)
1) Fruit	1) Vegetables	1) Fruit
2) Vegetables	2) Fruit	2) Vegetables
3) Whole grains	3) Nuts and soy protein	3) Nuts and legumes
4) Dairy	4) High white to red meat ratio	4) Whole grain
5) Total protein foods	5) Cereal fiber	5) Low-fat dairy
6) High poly- and monounsaturated fat to saturated fat ratio	6) No trans fat	6) Low sodium
7) Less refined grains	7) High polyunsaturated to saturated fat ratio	7) Less red and processed meats
8) Less sodium	8) Longer duration of multivitamin use	8) No sugar-sweetened beverages
9) Less added sugars	9) Moderate alcohol	
10) Less saturated fats	10) More variety	

Data from Morze J, Danielewicz A, Hoffmann G, Schwingshackl L. Diet Quality as Assessed by the Healthy Eating Index, Alternate Healthy Eating Index, Dietary Approaches to Stop Hypertension Score, and Health Outcomes: A Second Update of a Systematic Review and Meta-Analysis of Cohort Studies. *J Acad Nutr Diet.* 2020;120(12):1998-2031.e15.

Progress: A Report of the Surgeon General,[29] cigarette smoking is also a major risk factor for diabetes.

The risk of developing diabetes is 30% to 40% higher for active smokers than for nonsmokers.[29] A systematic review published as the Surgeon General's report reveals that, compared with people who have never smoked, the relative risk (RR) of developing type 2 diabetes is 1.37 for current smokers, 1.14 for former smokers, and 1.22 for passive smokers.[30] There are several biological mechanisms that explain the association between smoking and diabetes (**Box 3**).

Other Environmental Factors

Other environmental factors that impact the pathogenesis of diabetes include sleep (duration and quality), noise and air pollution, sedentary time, depression, socioeconomic factors, and arsenic exposure.

There is a U-shaped dose–response relationship between sleep duration and the risk of type 2 diabetes. The lowest risk of diabetes was observed with 7 to 8 hours of sleep per day. The relative risk (RR) for diabetes increased by 1.09 for each hour less of sleep for those who slept a total of less than 7 hours per day; and 1.14 for each additional hour of sleep for those who slept more than 8 hours.[34] Poor sleep quality (defined as difficulty falling asleep, difficulty staying asleep, or early morning arousal) is also associated with an increased risk of prediabetes and diabetes (RR of 1.31 and 1.30, respectively).[35]

Residential noise exposure is correlated with an increased incidence of diabetes; exposure to 60 to 70 dB versus less than 60 dB is associated with a 19% higher risk of diabetes. This is biologically plausible, as noise is a stressor that increases cortisol levels and insulin resistance. Residential noise also leads to disrupted sleep.[36] Long term exposure to air pollution and fine particulate matter is also correlated with metabolic syndrome and type 2 diabetes in adults.[37,38]

Sedentary behavior (sitting) seems to be an independent risk factor for diabetes. Both reducing and breaking up sitting time may be a useful strategy to prevent diabetes.[39] Television viewing time has been used as a surrogate for sedentary time. Those with high daily TV viewing time have a 1.12 RR of diabetes, compared with those with low TV viewing time.[40]

Depression has been recognized as a risk factor for diabetes, and diabetes is a risk factor for depression. Patients have worse metabolic control when depression and diabetes coexist.[41] Current Major Depressive Disorder (MDD) is associated with

---

Box 3
Biologic mechanisms linking smoking and diabetes

Smoking is associated with central obesity (increased ectopic fat).[29]

Smoking increases inflammation leading to insulin resistance.[31]

Smoking increases oxidative stress leading to insulin resistance.[29]

Pancreatic islet and beta-cells have nicotine receptors, and insulin release is reduced with exposure to nicotine.[32]

Smoking decreases the expression of peroxisome proliferator-activated receptor-gamma (PPAR-gamma), a transcription factor that promotes insulin sensitivity.[31]

Smoking increases blood arsenic levels.[31]

Smoking impacts insulin sensitivity through epigenetic factors, affecting 95 different DNA methylation sites.[31,33]

insulin resistance (OR 1.51), but remitted depression is not, suggesting that insulin resistance exists during depression but is not a biomarker for depression.[42]

Social determinants of health (SDoH) are environmental conditions that affect health outcomes and risks.[43] There is an association between childhood socioeconomic inequalities and the risk of type 2 diabetes later in life.[44] Compared with high levels of education, occupation, and income; low levels were associated with an increased risk of diabetes (RR 1.41, 1.31, and 1.40, respectively).[45] Education level and socioeconomic factors may not have a direct biological effect on disease—their effect is mediated mainly by smoking, obesity, chronic stress, and physical inactivity.[46]

Many cross-sectional studies have shown a dose-dependent relationship between arsenic exposure and diabetes.[47] Rice accumulates more arsenic than other food crops and is the biggest food source of inorganic arsenic.[48] This may explain why rice is so diabetogenic.

COVID-19

Viral infections have been widely associated with type 1 diabetes pathogenesis. A relationship between coronaviruses and diabetes was seen with the SARS-CoV pandemic of 2003.[49] Diabetic ketoacidosis (DKA) and hyperosmolar hyperglycemic states (HHS) are unusually common in patients with COVID-19 when compared with other equally critically ill patients. In a meta-analysis, 14.4% of hospitalized patients with COVID-19 are newly diagnosed with diabetes.[50] New-onset diabetes, DKA, and HHS are COVID-related conditions.

LIFESTYLE INTERVENTIONS
Preventing Progression of Prediabetes

Lifestyle interventions prevent the progression from prediabetes to diabetes. Because prediabetes frequently results in diabetes, the 2020 American Diabetes Association (ADA) Standards of Medical Care recommends annual screening for prediabetes in patients with the following risk factors: those who have a first degree relative with diabetes; a high-risk ethnicity (eg, African American, Latino, Native American, Asian American, Pacific Islander); a history of cardiovascular disease, hypertension, or lipid abnormalities; polycystic ovary syndrome (PCOS); physical inactivity; or other clinical conditions associated with insulin resistance (eg, severe obesity, acanthosis nigricans). Women who have ever been diagnosed with gestational diabetes should have lifelong testing for prediabetes at least every 3 years.[18]

Diabetes Prevention Program

Major trials in the United States,[51] Finland,[52] and in China[53,54] demonstrate that lifestyle interventions are highly effective in preventing type 2 diabetes. The Diabetes Prevention Program (DPP) in the United States showed that compared with standard lifestyle recommendations, intensive lifestyle intervention (**Box 4**) reduces the incidence of type 2 diabetes in patients with prediabetes by 58% in 2.8 years. A follow-up study showed a 34% reduction at 10 years.[55] Similar sustained incident diabetes reduction was seen in Finland and China.

The 2 major goals of the DPP lifestyle intervention were at least 7% weight loss and a minimum of 150 minutes of moderate-intensity physical activity per week. Weight loss was the most important factor to reduce the risk of incident diabetes. The initial focus was on reducing total fat rather than calories. After several weeks, the need to restrict calories was introduced. Weight loss was achieved by calculating calorie

---

Box 4
DPP intensive lifestyle intervention

Weight loss:
- $\geq$7% of initial weight in the first 6 months
- Pace: 1 to 2 pounds/wk
- Maintained throughout trial

Physical activity goal:
- 150 minutes of moderate physical activity distributed throughout the week
- Brisk walking stressed
- Alternatives (eg, aerobic dance, bicycling, skating, swimming) discussed
- Minimum 3 times per week, 10 minutes per session
- Maximum 75 minutes of strength training could be applied to goal
- Lifestyle activities (eg, stairs, stretching, gardening) were discussed but not part of goal
- Supervised physical activity available at least two times per week throughout the trial

Individual case managers:
- Each participant was assigned a "lifestyle coach"
- Most coaches were registered dietitians
- Some coaches had Master's degrees in exercise physiology, behavioral psychology, or health education
- Ratio of 1.5 to 2 coaches/40 participants

Curriculum:
- 16 Core sessions in the first 24 weeks
- Maintenance visits every 2 months for the remainder of the trial
- Phone contact at least once between maintenance visits
- Supplemental group classes, motivational campaigns, restart opportunities
- "Toolbox" of adherence strategies

Data from Diabetes Prevention Program (DPP) Research Group. The Diabetes Prevention Program (DPP): description of lifestyle intervention. *Diabetes Care*. 2002;25(12):2165-2171.

---

goals based on weight and subtracting 500 to 1000 calories per day. Weight loss drugs were not used in the study.

Even without weight loss, 150 minutes of physical activity per week (approximate 700 kcal per week energy expenditure) reduced the incidence of type 2 diabetes by 44%.[56] Participants exercised for a minimum of three times per week, and for at least 10 minutes per session with a maximum of 75 minutes of strength training applied toward the 150 minutes per week goal.[57]

The DPP intervention used an individual model of treatment, rather than a group-based approach. A 16-session core curriculum was completed within the first 24 weeks of the program. This was followed by face-to-face follow-up visits at least once every 2 months for the remainder of the trial, with phone check-ins between visits.

Support

To implement the lifestyle interventions used in the DPP study, the Centers for Disease Control and Prevention (CDC) developed the National Diabetes Prevention Program (National DPP) (www.cdc.gov/diabetes/prevention/index.htm).[58] Results from the CDC's National DPP during the first 4 years of implementation were promising: more than 35,000 people at high risk participated, 87% of participants attended at least 4 sessions, and more than half attended at least 14 sessions. Unfortunately, less than half attended the program for at least 6 months, and only 1 in 10 completed the full 22-session program.[59] Completing the program was especially difficult for individuals who were younger, and for members of racial or ethnic minority populations.

Other approaches to improve the implementation of lifestyle interventions may also be appropriate based on patient preferences and availability. The use of community health workers may facilitate the adoption of lifestyle behavior changes.[60] Registered dietitians (RDN) can also help individuals with prediabetes reach their diet and weight loss.[61] Pharmacists[62] and psychologists[63] can also be instrumental in achieving lifestyle and behavioral change.

SUMMARY

There are many nonmodifiable and modifiable risk factors for type 2 diabetes. Nonmodifiable risk factors include age, genetics, epigenetics, and social determinants of health (including education level, socioeconomic status, and noise and arsenic exposure). Modifiable risk factors include obesity, the gut microbiome, diet, cigarette smoking, sleep duration, sleep quality, and sedentary behavior. Major lifestyle interventions to prevent and treat diabetes relate to these risk factors. Weight loss is the lifestyle intervention with the largest benefit for both preventing and treating diabetes. Exercise, even without weight loss, significantly reduces the incidence of type 2 diabetes.

CLINICS CARE POINTS

- Always consider the possibility of diabetes when caring for obese patients, especially when the patients have central obesity and fatty liver
- Diabetes can be passed on genetically and epigenetically, so be mindful of maternal history of both diabetes and gestational diabetes
- Animal-based diets, when compared with plant-based diets, are associated with diabetes
- The Mediterranean diet significantly reduces diabetes risk, even without weight loss
- In addition to all the other things it causes, cigarette smoking is a major risk factor for diabetes
- Lifestyle interventions, especially weight loss, can prevent the progression of prediabetes to diabetes

CONFLICTS OF INTEREST

The author has nothing to disclose.

REFERENCES

1. NCD Risk Factor Collaboration (NCD-RisC). Worldwide trends in diabetes since 1980: a pooled analysis of 751 population-based studies with 4.4 million participants. Lancet 2016;387(10027):1513–30. https://doi.org/10.1016/S0140-6736(16)00618-8.
2. Kirkman MS, Briscoe VJ, Clark N, et al. Diabetes in older adults. Diabetes Care 2012;35(12):2650–64. https://doi.org/10.2337/dc12-1801.
3. Kalra S. Diabesity. J Pak Med Assoc 2013;63(4):532–4.
4. Chan JM, Rimm EB, Colditz GA, et al. Obesity, fat distribution, and weight gain as risk factors for clinical diabetes in men. Diabetes Care 1994;17(9):961–9. https://doi.org/10.2337/diacare.17.9.961.
5. Snel M, Jonker JT, Schoones J, et al. Ectopic fat and insulin resistance: pathophysiology and effect of diet and lifestyle interventions. Int J Endocrinol 2012; 2012:983814. https://doi.org/10.1155/2012/983814.

6. Sattar N, Gill JMR. Type 2 diabetes as a disease of ectopic fat? BMC Med 2014; 12:123. https://doi.org/10.1186/s12916-014-0123-4.

7. Huang-Doran I, Sleigh A, Rochford JJ, et al. Lipodystrophy: metabolic insights from a rare disorder. J Endocrinol 2010;207(3):245–55. https://doi.org/10.1677/JOE-10-0272.

8. Cleland SJ, Sattar N. Impact of ethnicity on metabolic disturbance, vascular dysfunction and atherothrombotic cardiovascular disease. Diabetes Obes Metab 2005;7(5):463–70. https://doi.org/10.1111/j.1463-1326.2004.00401.x.

9. McCarthy MI, Zeggini E. Genome-wide association studies in type 2 diabetes. Curr Diab Rep 2009;9(2):164–71. https://doi.org/10.1007/s11892-009-0027-4.

10. Chatterjee S, Khunti K, Davies MJ. Type 2 diabetes. Lancet 2017;389(10085): 2239–51. https://doi.org/10.1016/S0140-6736(17)30058-2.

11. Sommese L, Zullo A, Mancini FP, et al. Clinical relevance of epigenetics in the onset and management of type 2 diabetes mellitus. Epigenetics 2017;12(6): 401–15. https://doi.org/10.1080/15592294.2016.1278097.

12. Epigenetics. National Jewish Health. Available at: https://www.nationaljewish.org/research-science/programs-depts/center-for-genes-environment-and-health/research/epigenetics. March 17, 2021.

13. Bansal A, Simmons RA. Epigenetics and developmental origins of diabetes: correlation or causation? Am J Physiol Endocrinol Metab 2018;315(1):E15–28. https://doi.org/10.1152/ajpendo.00424.2017.

14. Vaiserman AM. Early-Life Nutritional Programming of Type 2 Diabetes: Experimental and Quasi-Experimental Evidence. Nutrients 2017;9(3). https://doi.org/10.3390/nu9030236.

15. Hales CN, Barker DJ, Clark PM, et al. Fetal and infant growth and impaired glucose tolerance at age 64. BMJ 1991;303(6809):1019–22.

16. David LA, Maurice CF, Carmody RN, et al. Diet rapidly and reproducibly alters the human gut microbiome. Nature 2014;505(7484):559–63. https://doi.org/10.1038/nature12820.

17. Caesar R. Pharmacologic and nonpharmacologic therapies for the gut microbiota in type 2 diabetes. Can J Diabetes 2019;43(3):224–31. https://doi.org/10.1016/j.jcjd.2019.01.007.

18. American Diabetes Association. 3. Prevention or Delay of Type 2 Diabetes: Standards of Medical Care in Diabetes-2021. Diabetes Care 2021;44(Suppl 1):S34–9. https://doi.org/10.2337/dc21-S003.

19. Ajala O, English P, Pinkney J. Systematic review and meta-analysis of different dietary approaches to the management of type 2 diabetes. Am J Clin Nutr 2013; 97(3):505–16. https://doi.org/10.3945/ajcn.112.042457.

20. Salas-Salvadó J, Bulló M, Babio N, et al. Reduction in the incidence of type 2 diabetes with the Mediterranean diet: results of the PREDIMED-Reus nutrition intervention randomized trial. Diabetes Care 2011;34(1):14–9. https://doi.org/10.2337/dc10-1288.

21. Golan R, Gepner Y, Shai I. Wine and Health-New Evidence. Eur J Clin Nutr 2019; 72(Suppl 1):55–9. https://doi.org/10.1038/s41430-018-0309-5.

22. Morze J, Danielewicz A, Hoffmann G, et al. Diet Quality as Assessed by the Healthy Eating Index, Alternate Healthy Eating Index, Dietary Approaches to Stop Hypertension Score, and Health Outcomes: A Second Update of a Systematic Review and Meta-Analysis of Cohort Studies. J Acad Nutr Diet 2020;120(12): 1998–2031.e15. https://doi.org/10.1016/j.jand.2020.08.076.

23. Lee Y, Park K. Adherence to a Vegetarian Diet and Diabetes Risk: A Systematic Review and Meta-Analysis of Observational Studies. Nutrients 2017;9(6). https://doi.org/10.3390/nu9060603.

24. Qian F, Liu G, Hu FB, et al. Association Between Plant-Based Dietary Patterns and Risk of Type 2 Diabetes: A Systematic Review and Meta-analysis. JAMA Intern Med 2019;179(10):1335–44. https://doi.org/10.1001/jamainternmed.2019.2195.

25. Schwingshackl L, Hoffmann G. Diet quality as assessed by the Healthy Eating Index, the Alternate Healthy Eating Index, the Dietary Approaches to Stop Hypertension score, and health outcomes: a systematic review and meta-analysis of cohort studies. J Acad Nutr Diet 2015;115(5):780–800.e5. https://doi.org/10.1016/j.jand.2014.12.009.

26. Butt MS, Sultan MT. Coffee and its consumption: benefits and risks. Crit Rev Food Sci Nutr 2011;51(4):363–73. https://doi.org/10.1080/10408390903586412.

27. Allen RW, Schwartzman E, Baker WL, et al. Cinnamon use in type 2 diabetes: an updated systematic review and meta-analysis. Ann Fam Med 2013;11(5):452–9. https://doi.org/10.1370/afm.1517.

28. Costello RB, Dwyer JT, Saldanha L, et al. Do cinnamon supplements have a role in glycemic control in type 2 diabetes? a narrative review. J Acad Nutr Diet 2016;116(11):1794–802. https://doi.org/10.1016/j.jand.2016.07.015.

29. US Department of Health and Human Services, Centers for Disease Control and Prevention. The health Consequences of smoking—50 Years of progress. A report of the Surgeon general. 2014. Available at: https://bookstore-gpo-gov.libproxy.lib.unc.edu/products/health-consequences-smoking-50-years-progress-report-surgeon-general-full-report-epub-ebook. March 17, 2021.

30. Pan A, Wang Y, Talaei M, et al. Relation of active, passive, and quitting smoking with incident type 2 diabetes: a systematic review and meta-analysis. Lancet Diabetes Endocrinol 2015;3(12):958–67. https://doi.org/10.1016/S2213-8587(15)00316-2.

31. Maddatu J, Anderson-Baucum E, Evans-Molina C. Smoking and the risk of type 2 diabetes. Transl Res 2017;184:101–7. https://doi.org/10.1016/j.trsl.2017.02.004.

32. Yoshikawa H, Hellström-Lindahl E, Grill V. Evidence for functional nicotinic receptors on pancreatic beta cells. Metab Clin Exp 2005;54(2):247–54. https://doi.org/10.1016/j.metabol.2004.08.020.

33. Lin W-Y, Liu Y-L, Yang AC, et al. Active cigarette smoking is associated with an exacerbation of genetic susceptibility to diabetes. Diabetes 2020;69(12):2819–29. https://doi.org/10.2337/db20-0156.

34. Shan Z, Ma H, Xie M, et al. Sleep duration and risk of type 2 diabetes: a meta-analysis of prospective studies. Diabetes Care 2015;38(3):529–37. https://doi.org/10.2337/dc14-2073.

35. Kowall B, Lehnich A-T, Strucksberg K-H, et al. Associations among sleep disturbances, nocturnal sleep duration, daytime napping, and incident prediabetes and type 2 diabetes: the Heinz Nixdorf Recall Study. Sleep Med 2016;21:35–41. https://doi.org/10.1016/j.sleep.2015.12.017.

36. Dzhambov AM. Long-term noise exposure and the risk for type 2 diabetes: a meta-analysis. Noise Health 2015;17(74):23–33. https://doi.org/10.4103/1463-1741.149571.

37. Eze IC, Schaffner E, Foraster M, et al. Long-Term Exposure to Ambient Air Pollution and Metabolic Syndrome in Adults. PLoS One 2015;10(6):e0130337. https://doi.org/10.1371/journal.pone.0130337.

38. Weinmayr G, Hennig F, Fuks K, et al. Long-term exposure to fine particulate matter and incidence of type 2 diabetes mellitus in a cohort study: effects of total and traffic-specific air pollution. Environ Health 2015;14:53. https://doi.org/10.1186/s12940-015-0031-x.
39. Dempsey PC, Grace MS, Dunstan DW. Adding exercise or subtracting sitting time for glycaemic control: where do we stand? Diabetologia 2017;60(3):390–4. https://doi.org/10.1007/s00125-016-4180-4.
40. Hamilton MT, Hamilton DG, Zderic TW. Sedentary behavior as a mediator of type 2 diabetes. Med Sport Sci 2014;60:11–26. https://doi.org/10.1159/000357332.
41. Réus GZ, Dos Santos MAB, Strassi AP, et al. Pathophysiological mechanisms involved in the relationship between diabetes and major depressive disorder. Life Sci 2017;183:78–82. https://doi.org/10.1016/j.lfs.2017.06.025.
42. Watson K, Nasca C, Aasly L, et al. Insulin resistance, an unmasked culprit in depressive disorders: Promises for interventions. Neuropharmacology 2018; 136(Pt B):327–34. https://doi.org/10.1016/j.neuropharm.2017.11.038.
43. Social determinants of health | healthy people 2020. Available at: https://www.healthypeople.gov/node/3499/2020/topics-objectives/topic/social-determinants-health. Accessed March 18, 2021.
44. Tamayo T, Christian H, Rathmann W. Impact of early psychosocial factors (childhood socioeconomic factors and adversities) on future risk of type 2 diabetes, metabolic disturbances and obesity: a systematic review. BMC Public Health 2010;10:525. https://doi.org/10.1186/1471-2458-10-525.
45. Agardh E, Allebeck P, Hallqvist J, et al. Type 2 diabetes incidence and socioeconomic position: a systematic review and meta-analysis. Int J Epidemiol 2011;40(3):804–18. https://doi.org/10.1093/ije/dyr029.
46. Sacerdote C, Ricceri F, Rolandsson O, et al. Lower educational level is a predictor of incident type 2 diabetes in European countries: the EPIC-InterAct study. Int J Epidemiol 2012;41(4):1162–73. https://doi.org/10.1093/ije/dys091.
47. Farkhondeh T, Samarghandian S, Azimi-Nezhad M. The role of arsenic in obesity and diabetes. J Cell Physiol 2019;234(8):12516–29. https://doi.org/10.1002/jcp.28112.
48. Arnarson A. Arsenic in Rice: Should You Be Concerned? Healthline. 2017. Available at: https://www.healthline.com/nutrition/arsenic-in-rice. March 18, 2021.
49. Caruso P, Longo M, Esposito K, et al. Type 1 diabetes triggered by covid-19 pandemic: A potential outbreak? Diabetes Res Clin Pract 2020;164:108219. https://doi.org/10.1016/j.diabres.2020.108219.
50. Sathish T, Kapoor N, Cao Y, et al. Proportion of newly diagnosed diabetes in COVID-19 patients: A systematic review and meta-analysis. Diabetes Obes Metab. 2021. 23(3):870-874. doi:10.1111/dom.14269
51. Knowler WC, Barrett-Connor E, Fowler SE, et al. Reduction in the incidence of type 2 diabetes with lifestyle intervention or metformin. N Engl J Med 2002; 346(6):393–403. https://doi.org/10.1056/NEJMoa012512.
52. Lindström J, Ilanne-Parikka P, Peltonen M, et al. Sustained reduction in the incidence of type 2 diabetes by lifestyle intervention: follow-up of the Finnish Diabetes Prevention Study. Lancet 2006;368(9548):1673–9. https://doi.org/10.1016/S0140-6736(06)69701-8.
53. Li G, Zhang P, Wang J, et al. Cardiovascular mortality, all-cause mortality, and diabetes incidence after lifestyle intervention for people with impaired glucose tolerance in the Da Qing Diabetes Prevention Study: a 23-year follow-up study. Lancet Diabetes Endocrinol 2014;2(6):474–80. https://doi.org/10.1016/S2213-8587(14)70057-9.

54. Gong Q, Zhang P, Wang J, et al. Morbidity and mortality after lifestyle intervention for people with impaired glucose tolerance: 30-year results of the Da Qing Diabetes Prevention Outcome Study. Lancet Diabetes Endocrinol 2019;7(6): 452–61. https://doi.org/10.1016/S2213-8587(19)30093-2.

55. Knowler WC, Fowler SE, Hamman RR, et al, Diabetes Prevention Program Research Group. 10-year follow-up of diabetes incidence and weight loss in the Diabetes Prevention Program Outcomes Study. Lancet 2009;374(9702): 1677–86. https://doi.org/10.1016/S0140-6736(09)61457-4.

56. Hamman RF, Wing RR, Edelstein SL, et al. Effect of weight loss with lifestyle intervention on risk of diabetes. Diabetes Care 2006;29(9):2102–7. https://doi.org/10.2337/dc06-0560.

57. Diabetes Prevention Program (DPP) Research Group. The Diabetes Prevention Program (DPP): description of lifestyle intervention. Diabetes Care 2002;25(12): 2165–71. https://doi.org/10.2337/diacare.25.12.2165.

58. Ely EK, Gruss SM, Luman ET, et al. A National Effort to Prevent Type 2 Diabetes: Participant-Level Evaluation of CDC's National Diabetes Prevention Program. Diabetes Care 2017;40(10):1331–41. https://doi.org/10.2337/dc16-2099.

59. Cannon MJ, Masalovich S, Ng BP, et al. Retention Among Participants in the National Diabetes Prevention Program Lifestyle Change Program, 2012-2017. Diabetes Care 2020;43(9):2042–9. https://doi.org/10.2337/dc19-2366.

60. Community Preventive Services Task Force. Tffrs - diabetes prevention: interventions Engaging community health workers. The community Guide. 2016. Available at: https://www.thecommunityguide.org/content/tffrs-diabetes-prevention-interventions-engaging-community-health-workers. March 15, 2021.

61. Briggs Early K, Stanley K. Position of the academy of nutrition and dietetics: the role of medical nutrition therapy and registered dietitian nutritionists in the prevention and treatment of prediabetes and type 2 diabetes. J Acad Nutr Diet 2018; 118(2):343–53. https://doi.org/10.1016/j.jand.2017.11.021.

62. Hudspeth BD. Power of prevention: the pharmacist's role in prediabetes management. Diabetes Spectr 2018;31(4):320–3. https://doi.org/10.2337/ds18-0021.

63. Hilliard ME, Powell PW, Anderson BJ. Evidence-based behavioral interventions to promote diabetes management in children, adolescents, and families. Am Psychol 2016;71(7):590–601. https://doi.org/10.1037/a0040359.

Glycemic Targets and Glucose Monitoring

Tamara K. Oser, MD[a], Sean M. Oser, MD, MPH[b],*

KEYWORDS

- A_{1c} • Self-monitoring of blood glucose • Continuous glucose monitoring • Glycemia
- Glycemic targets • Hypoglycemia • Glucose management indicator • GMI

KEY POINTS

- Glucose monitoring is an important part of diabetes management.
- Periodic assessment of glycemia over a period of time is recommended for all individuals with diabetes. Methods to do this include measurement of glycated hemoglobin A_{1c}, continuous glucose monitoring (CGM), fructosamine, and glycated albumin.
- With the advent of CGM, additional insights into glycemia and patterns are attainable and may be valuable additions. CGM metrics provide information not only on overall glycemia but also on hypoglycemia, hyperglycemia, and glycemic variability, which can each be assessed and addressed therapeutically.
- Although targets for measures of glycemia may be individually determined by factors specific to a patient and/or their provider, most glycemic targets have been standardized.
- Most patients with type 1 diabetes or type 2 diabetes have the following recommended glycemic targets: A1c <7.0%, Glucose Management Indicator <7.0%, Time-In-Range (70-180mg/dL) >70%, Time-Below-Range (<70mg/dL) <4%, Time-Below-Range (<54%) <1%, Glycemic Variability ≥36%.

Monitoring glycemia is considered a cornerstone of diabetes care, and results are used to adjust therapies, to understand the impact of diet and exercise on glucose, and to stratify risk—especially as high glucose and low glucose increase the risk of a host of other potential complications. Glycemic monitoring includes patient self-monitoring as well as office-based and laboratory-based methods and has rapidly advanced since 1908, when the first copper reagent for urine glucose was developed.[1] The primary focus of this article is to review the history of glucose monitoring and current glycemic targets and monitoring in type 1 diabetes (T1D) and type 2 diabetes (T2D).

[a] Primary Care Diabetes Lab and High Plains Research Network, Department of Family Medicine, University of Colorado School of Medicine, 12631 East 17th, Avenue, Box F496, Aurora, CO 80045, USA; [b] Practice Innovation Program of Colorado, Primary Care Diabetes Lab, and UCHealth Lone Tree Primary Care, Department of Family Medicine, University of Colorado School of Medicine, 12631 East 17th Avenue, Box F496, Aurora, CO 80045, USA
* Corresponding author.
E-mail address: sean.oser@cuanschutz.edu

Prim Care Clin Office Pract 49 (2022) 213–223
https://doi.org/10.1016/j.pop.2021.11.002
0095-4543/22/© 2021 Elsevier Inc. All rights reserved.

HISTORY OF GLUCOSE MONITORING

In 1674, Thomas Willis was the first known Western doctor to taste urine and connect the sweetness of urine to the condition of the patient.[2] He did not figure out why this was so, but he added the term "mellitus"—Latin for honeyed or sweet—to "diabetes." His observations helped future researchers characterize diabetes mellitus and the finding of glucose in the urine of affected individuals.[3] Urine testing methods became a key way to determine whether someone had diabetes mellitus, with various methods described in a lecture printed in an 1884 edition of the *British Medical Journal*.[4] Among people with diabetes, assessing for the presence or absence of glucose in urine became and remained the standard method for determining diabetes status well into the twentieth century, with people mixing urine with reagents like Benedict solution and boiling the mixtures in glass vessels routinely, often daily.

However, in 1965, Ames developed the first blood glucose testing strip, which used a large blood sample and was only available in physician offices.[5] By 1980, blood glucose meters became available, and over the next 2 decades became smaller, required less blood, decreased in cost, and demonstrated improved accuracy. Self-monitoring of blood glucose (SMBG) became the standard of care, especially for patients with T1D. Early SMBG systems required a drop of blood to react with a test strip for 60 seconds, to be wiped off, and then to "develop" for 60 seconds before the meter read a color change on the strip and displayed a result. SMBG systems evolved further, requiring less time to react and to develop, and eventually not requiring the wiping of the blood drop at all. Sixty seconds became 45 seconds, then 30 seconds, then 15 seconds, and finally, 10 seconds, 6 seconds, and even just 5 seconds to see a result. By 2010, SMBG was recommended for all patients receiving insulin.[5]

Glucose monitoring was further revolutionized with the introduction of continuous glucose monitoring (CGM). In 1999, the first professional CGM was approved by the Food and Drug Administration, where blinded glucose data were collected from the patient for 3 days, and the information was downloaded for the health care provider to review. CGM technology has continued to evolve relatively quickly since 1999 (**Fig. 1**), and CGM can now offer the ability to provide real-time data to patients and to do so without finger sticks. The accuracy of CGM has also continued to improve, as measured by the mean absolute relative difference (MARD), which indicates the average discrepancy between a given system's results and gold-standard reference values, where MARD $\leq 10\%$ is considered sufficiently accurate to inform insulin dosing decisions.[6] Current CGM systems have achieved MARD less than 10% and are approximately as accurate as most SMBG meters.[7,8]

As glucose assessment techniques evolved, evidence also mounted for the importance of maintaining blood glucose as close to normal as possible, minimizing hyperglycemia to reduce risk of long-term complications, minimizing hypoglycemia to reduce risk of shorter-term adverse events and longer-term complications, and minimizing glucose variability for many of the same reasons. As such, short-, intermediate-, and longer-term measures of glycemia have become central to diabetes management, as have glycemia targets associated with these various modes of glycemia assessment.

DISCUSSION: PRESENT DAY GLUCOSE MONITORING

Broadly speaking, glucose monitoring can occur at the laboratory level or at the patient level, with multiple approaches available in each context. With increasing frequency, some laboratory-based assessments are available as point-of-care assessments in clinical settings, like an office-based practice. The various contexts and assessment methods are reviewed in later discussion.

CGM Accuracy: MARD (Mean Absolute Relative Difference)

2005	Medtronic RT-Guardian	19.7%
	Abbott FreeStyle Navigator	12.8%
	Medtronic RT-CGM	15.8%
	Dexcom SEVEN Plus	15.9%
	Medtronic Enlite	13.8%
	Dexcom G4 Platinum	13.0%
	Dexcom G4 Platinum w/505	9.0%
	Dexcom G5	9.0%
	Dexcom G6	9.0%
	Medtronic Guardian 3	8.7–10.6%
	Freestyle Libre 10 d	9.7%
	Eversense CGM	9.4%
2020	Freestyle Libre 14 d	9.4%

Fig. 1. MARD of various CGM systems from 2005 to 2020. MARD is a measure of accuracy, with MARD $\leq$10% considered sufficiently accurate to allow therapeutic/medication of dosing decisions. MARD data presented here compiled from numerous sources.[9–17]

Laboratory and Point-of-care Based Assessment

Hemoglobin A_{1c}

Glycemic control can be assessed through glycated hemoglobin A_{1c} (A_{1c}), which reflects average glycemia over approximately 3 months. To date, most existing clinical trials use A_{1c} as the metric for glycemia, and it has strong predictive value for diabetes complications.[18–20] A_{1c} has been the predominantly standard approach to glycemia assessment for many years now. A_{1c} testing assesses the proportion of hemoglobin A_{1c} that is glycosylated (has glucose attached permanently, for the life of the red blood cell to which it is attached), reported traditionally in the United States as a percentage. A_{1c} is positively associated with average glucose over the preceding 3 months; the higher the A_{1c} level, the higher the average glucose. Frequency of A_{1c} assessment depends on factors including clinician judgment and treatment regimen, and A_{1c} testing only twice per year may be adequate for patients with T2D with stable glucose control. However, patients on intensive insulin regimens or not at goal A_{1c} may require assessment more frequently. The American Diabetes Association (ADA) Standards of Medical Care recommends assessing glycemic status at least 2 times a year in people who are meeting treatment goals and have stable glycemic control. They recommend more frequent assessment (at least quarterly and additional assessments at the clinician's discretion) for those who have had a recent change in therapy and/or who are not achieving glycemic targets.[21]

Fructosamine and Glycated Albumin

Some patient populations (eg, patients with red blood cell disorders, patients with renal disease, and others) will have inaccurate or unreliable results from assessing A_{1c}. Fructosamine assessment may be an alternative to A_{1c} in assessing glycemia in these populations, as may glycated albumin. Fructosamine and glycated albumin assessment can provide information on average glycemia over approximately the preceding 2 weeks, in contrast to the roughly 3-month view offered by A_{1c} assessment. Like A_{1c}, they are positively associated with average glucose concentration.

Serum Glucose

Serum glucose assessment can also be assessed at the laboratory and/or point-of-care level and is done so quite frequently, often as part of a metabolic profile or panel. It indicates glucose concentration at the moment of the blood draw and is not a summary indicator of average glycemia as are the other methods mentioned earlier. Interpretation of results generally depends on whether the patient was fasting (no caloric intake for at least several hours before acquiring the blood sample) or not. It is also routinely used as a component of other testing protocols, such as oral glucose challenge testing, which involves serial serum glucose concentration assessment.

Patient Level Assessment

Hemoglobin A$_{1c}$

Although traditionally assessed in the laboratory or at the point-of-care, home A$_{1c}$ kits are available through retail pharmacies, online vendors, and mail-in laboratories with self-collection. Although such use may expand in the future, laboratory testing and point-of-care assessment of A$_{1c}$ still predominate.

Self-Monitoring of Blood Glucose

SMBG involves individual capillary glucose level determination, usually from the finger, although alternate site testing has become an option as well. Like serum glucose assessment in the laboratory, SMBG provides a momentary assessment of glucose concentration. Repeated measurements may provide additional context, for example, at different times of day, or at the same time of day on repeated days. Numerous glucose meter products from numerous manufacturers are available, and they tend to have in common the need to obtain a capillary blood sample (generally 1 small drop, although the size or volume varies somewhat) using a lancet, a strip to which the sample is applied, and the meter to measure the glucose concentration. The measurement systems generally rely on the blood sample interacting with glucose oxidase on the strip, allowing the meter to measure the results of this reaction and express a blood glucose concentration. Frequency of SMBG, or even whether SMBG is recommended at all, depends on multiple factors. One such factor is the patient's diabetes type, as frequent SMBG checks (4 or more per day, every day) are routinely recommended for people with T1D and may be recommended for people with T2D who use multiple daily injections or continuous infusion of insulin. Other factors might include patient-specific experience, with more frequent checks perhaps recommended for those who experience frequent hypoglycemia, hyperglycemia, or glucose fluctuation, whereas some may be recommended to check their glucose by SMBG just once per day, or not at all. Still, other factors might include medication regimen, provider preference, patient preference, and patient resources.

Continuous Glucose Monitoring

Generally based on glucose oxidase (like conventional SMBG strips), CGM provides "continuous" measurements. Depending on the product, the frequency can vary from every 15 minutes to every 1 minute and is often every 5 minutes. This provides up to 96 readings per day (every 15 minutes), 288 readings per day (every 5 minutes), or 1440 readings per day (every 1 minute). Any given reading reflects the glucose concentration of the interstitial fluid at that moment (closely related to blood glucose concentration), much the same as SMBG does. However, the continuous measurements and software capabilities of CGM systems lead to numerous other capabilities as well, including the ability to potentially detect hypoglycemia earlier, when less severe or when presymptomatic, or even to predict impending hypoglycemia, allowing an opportunity to avert it altogether. Earlier intervention leads to less frequent hypoglycemia, shorter duration of hypoglycemia, and lower severity of hypoglycemia. CGM systems also display glucose trend—which direction the glucose is headed right now. It may be particularly useful to know not just that the glucose, for example, at bedtime, is 110 mg/dL as with SMBG, but whether it is 110 mg/dL and stable, 110 mg/dL and falling (and whether it is falling slowly, moderately, or quickly), or 110 mg/dL and rising (again, slowly, moderately, or quickly). This added information about which direction the glucose is headed can lead to very different decisions about what to do with such a glucose level (and direction) at bedtime. The added data and its visualization on reader devices, smart-phones, smartwatches, and tablet/computer devices can bring new insights that are diffi-cult to discern with less data and less visualization. This can be likened to the ability to learn more and to gain further insight from a movie than from a series of photographs or a single photograph. As depicted in **Fig. 2**, for example, a daily fingerstick SMBG reading provides just 1 data point, but one has no real ability to discern how a patient's glucose levels might vary until the next reading, say the next day. Likewise, a few readings in a day may add more detail, but much less so than the continuous tracing one can see from readings every few minutes. The continuous glucose data can reveal otherwise un-detectable incidents and even patterns of high-glucose readings and/or low-glucose readings that the other methods are more likely to miss.

Other capabilities that become available with this continuous stream of data include new metrics that are not available with conventional SMBG. For example, CGM sys-tems can calculate and report the average glucose level recorded from the sensor readings and can also convert this into the Glucose Management Indicator (GMI), a metric analogous to the A_{1c}, but for user- or provider-specified intervals, such as 14 days, 30 days, 90 days, and so forth, whereas A_{1c} is limited to roughly a 2- to 3-month look-back. Also, in contrast to A_{1c}, GMI (and other CGM metrics) is not subject to racial/ethnic and other genetic or health condition-related factors that can make A_{1c} unreliable and/or inaccurate; examples include the observed differences in A_{1c} mea-surement between black and white individuals as well as the falsely elevated or falsely lowered results that can be seen with hemoglobinopathies, anemias, renal disease, pregnancy, and other conditions.[22]

Continuous Glucose Monitoring Metrics. In addition to GMI, there are other CGM metrics that can be quite useful in providing greater insights into glycemia and its pat-terns in an individual. GMI, like A_{1c}, reflects average glycemia, without insight into glucose fluctuation or variability. However, glucose variability is increasingly associ-ated with risk of mortality, cardiovascular disease, cognitive impairment, and lower

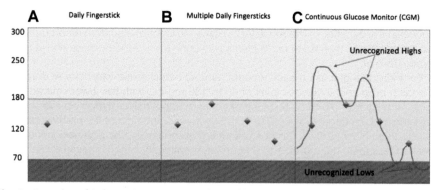

Fig. 2. Quantity of information, patterns observable, and events identifiable by (A) once daily SMBG, (B) multiple daily glucose checks via SMBG, and (C) CGM.

quality of life. CGM systems can measure and calculate glycemic variability (GV) and can thereby inform therapeutic approaches to manage GV. The utility of this metric can be appreciated when considering 2 patients with equivalent A_{1c} results: 1 patient experiences very little hyperglycemia and very little hypoglycemia, with their readings relatively steady (and therefore with little variability), whereas the other patient experiences dramatic hyperglycemia and hypoglycemia with tremendous fluctuation around the mean glucose shared with the other patient (but therefore with high GV). With A_{1c} alone, the differences between these 2 patients' glycemic patterns would be impossible to discern, whereas CGM and its ability to provide GV information reveal stark differences between these two. In addition to GMI and GV, CGM systems can provide information on time spent in various glycemic ranges, including time-in-range (TIR), time-below-range (TBR), and time-above-range (TAR). Each of these provides somewhat different and more information than the other metrics already mentioned and rounds out the picture of near-euglycemia, hypoglycemia, and hyperglycemia, respectively. International consensus has standardized both the ranges themselves and the targets for time spent in those ranges, which are summarized in **Table 1**.

GLYCEMIC TARGETS

As the available methods of assessing and monitoring glucose have changed over time, the recommended targets for each of these have evolved as well. Glycemic targets for various assessment methods are summarized in **Table 2**.

A_{1c} targets have received perhaps the most attention, as A_{1c} has dominated most of the past 3 decades as the most used and most researched glycemic indicator. A_{1c} targets vary from 1 specialty association to another, and often from 1 patient population to another. For most nonpregnant patients with diabetes, the ADA,[21] Diabetes Canada (DC),[23] and others recommend an A_{1c} goal of less than 7.0%. Other more and less stringent examples exist, with the American College of Physicians recommending an A_{1c} target of 7% to 8% for most people with diabetes,[24] whereas the American Association of Clinical Endocrinologists (AACE) and the American College of Endocrinology (ACE) recommend for most that the "optimal A_{1c} is $\leq$ 6.5%, or as close to normal as is safe and achievable."[25] Other variations also exist, for example, with the ADA stating the acceptability and potential benefit of a lower A_{1c} goal per patient and provider preference if such a level can be safely achieved (noting the potential safety risks of hypoglycemia or other adverse events).[21] Likewise, the ADA states that "less stringent" A_{1c} goals may be appropriate for some patients, such as those with limited life expectancy or for whom the harms of treatment to a lower target might outweigh the benefits.[21] The AACE/ACE Glycemic Control Algorithm recommends an A_{1c} target greater than 6.5% for "patients with concurrent serious illness and at risk for hypoglycemia."[25]

For individual glucose measurements, targets can likewise vary. The ADA recommends a preprandial glucose level of 80 to 130 mg/dL, with the lower limit adjusted fairly recently from 70 to 80 because of concern about risk of hypoglycemia with the lower limit of the target range.[21] The AACE/ACE recommendation for premeal glucose is less than 110 mg/dL.[25] For postprandial glucose levels, the ADA recommends a peak of less than 180 mg/dL 1 to 2 hours after eating.[21]

The ADA also recommends revisiting and raising glycemic targets for individuals who are treated with insulin and who have hypoglycemia unawareness, 1 episode of level 3 hypoglycemia (a severe event involving altered mental and/or physical function, requiring assistance from another person for recovery), or repeated unexplained

Table 1
Glycemic metrics and targets for most people with diabetes (including type 1 diabetes and type 2 diabetes)

Metric	Method of Assessing	Description	Target for Most People with Diabetes
A_{1c}	Blood (laboratory, point-of-care, or home kit)	Percentage of hemoglobin A_{1c} that is glycosylated, reflecting average glycemia	Individualized, but generally: <7.0% (ADA, DC) or ≤6.5% (AACE/ACE) or 7.0%–8.0% (ACP)
Preprandial glucose	Blood (laboratory, point-of-care, or SMBG)	Blood glucose level assessed before eating (eg, before meal, fasting)	Individualized, but generally: 80–130 mg/dL (ADA) or <110 mg/dL (AACE/ACE)
Postprandial glucose	Blood (laboratory, point-of-care, or SMBG)	Blood glucose level assessed after eating, generally 1–2 h later	
Average glucose	CGM, SMBG	Mean of glucose readings from CGM or from SMBG (if multiple daily SMBG readings are obtained; typically at least 6 per day)	Depends on A_{1c} target; generally: <154 mg/dL (ADA, DC) or ≤140 mg/dL (AACE/ACE) or 154–183 mg/dL (ACP)
GMI	CGM	Reflection of average glycemia, calculated from average glucose to be expressed in the same units as A_{1c} (%) and therefore allowing comparison to A_{1c}	Depends on A_{1c} target; generally: <7.0% (ADA) or ≤6.5% (AACE/ACE) or 7.0%–8.0% (ACP)
TIR	CGM	TIR; percentage of sensor readings between 70 and 180 mg/dL	>70%
TBR <70	CGM	Percentage of sensor readings <70 mg/dL	<4%
TBR <54	CGM	Percentage of sensor readings <54 mg/dL	<1%
TAR >180	CGM	Percentage of sensor readings >180 mg/dL	<25%
TAR >250	CGM	Percentage of sensor readings >250 mg/dL	<5%
GV	CGM	GV (%CV); standard deviation of sensor readings divided by mean of sensor readings	≤36%

Abbreviations: %CV, percent coefficient of variation; ACP, American College of Physicians.
  Data from Refs.[21],[23–26]

level 2 hypoglycemia (glucose level <54 mg/dL).[21] They recommend that the increase in glycemic targets be maintained for at least several weeks, in order to allow at least partial reversal of hypoglycemia unawareness and reduction of risk of recurrent episodes of hypoglycemia.

Table 2
Glycemic metrics and specialized targets for specific populations of people with diabetes

		Target Range *Goal*	
Metric	Older/high-risk patients with T1D or T1D	Pregnancy with T1D	Gestational diabetes or pregnancy with T2D
A_{1c}	Personalize target	<6% if safely achievable, or <7% if necessary to prevent hypoglycemia	<6% if safely achievable, or <7% if necessary to prevent hypoglycemia
Preprandial glucose	80–130 mg/dL (for older but healthy individuals) 90–150 mg/dL (for more complex health status) 100–150 mg/dL (for very complex, cognitive impairment, or limited life expectancy)	<95 mg/dL	<95 mg/dL
Postprandial glucose			
1-h postprandial	n/a	<140 mg/dL	<140 mg/dL
2-h postprandial	n/a	<120 mg/dL	<120 mg/dL
Bedtime glucose	80–180 mg/dL (for older but healthy individuals) 100–180 mg/dL (for more complex health status) 110–200 mg/dL (for very complex, limited life expectancy)		
Average glucose	Personalize target	Use as adjunct to SMBG and A_{1c} in pregnancy	Use as adjunct to SMBG and A_{1c} in pregnancy
GMI	Personalize target	Should not be used in pregnancy as an A_{1c} estimate	Should not be used in pregnancy as an A_{1c} estimate
TIR	70–180 mg/dL >50%	63–140 mg/dL >70%	63–140 mg/dL *Not yet determined*
TBR level 1 + level 2	<70 mg/dL <1%	<63 mg/dL <4%	<63 mg/dL *Not yet determined*
TBR level 2	n/a	<54 mg/dL <1%	<54 mg/dL *Not yet determined*
TAR level 1 + level 2	n/a	>140 mg/dL <25%	>140 mg/dL *Not yet determined*
TAR level 2	>250 mg/dL <10%	n/a	n/a

Abbreviation: n/a, not applicable.
  Data from Refs.[21,24–26]

Moving on to CGM glycemic targets, this area has become much more robust, with a corresponding growth in recognition of how useful CGM can be. Because of the range of complementary but distinct ways to gauge glycemia using CGM metrics, it is quite helpful that there is international consensus on which CGM metrics are most useful clinically, what their definitions are, and in most cases what their targets should be. The numerous specialty organizations that have drafted and endorsed this standardization include the ADA, AACE, Association of Diabetes Care and Education Specialists (formerly the American Association of Diabetes Educators), the European Association for the Study of Diabetes, the Foundation of European Nurses in Diabetes, the International Society for Pediatric and Adolescent Diabetes, JDRF, and the Pediatric Endocrine Society.[26] For some metrics, there is no standard target (eg, the GMI, which approximates and can be a surrogate for A_{1c}, which itself has varying target levels recommended, depending on individual patient circumstances). For most, though, recommended targets are made for 2 broad groups: (1) most people with T1D or T2D; and (2) older and/or high-risk individuals with T1D or T2D. Notably, different targets exist for others, especially for those with diabetes in pregnancy. The metrics and targets are detailed in **Tables 1 and 2**.

SUMMARY

Glycemic monitoring has changed dramatically over recent decades. Assessing glycemia over a period of time remains a standard recommendation in the care of all people with diabetes. Methods for assessing glycemia range from laboratory of office-based methods to patient-based methods. Assessing A_{1c} has been the most common method of assessing overall glycemia for a long time. CGM can also be used to assess overall glycemia, especially via GMI and/or TIR, which can be useful especially when A_{1c} might be unreliable or inaccurate, or when such information is desired to reflect a measurement time of less than 3 months. Other measures of glycemia, including hypoglycemia and GV, are becoming increasingly important in some cases and are also available via CGM. For most people with diabetes, glycemic targets have been standardized, with some variation in recommendations about A_{1c}, but with international consensus on CGM metrics like TIR, TBR, TAR, and GV.

CLINICS CARE POINTS

- Glucose monitoring is an important part of diabetes management.
- Periodic assessment of glycemia over a period of time is recommended for all individuals with diabetes. Methods to do this include measurement of glycated hemoglobin A_{1c}, continuous glucose monitoring, fructosamine, and glycated albumin.
- With the advent of continuous glucose monitoring, additional insights into glycemia and patterns are attainable and may be valuable additions. Continuous glucose monitoring metrics provide information not only on overall glycemia but also on hypoglycemia, hyperglycemia, and glycemic variability, which can each be assessed and addressed therapeutically.
- Although targets for measures of glycemia may be individually determined by factors specific to a patient and/or their provider, most glycemic targets have been standardized.
- Most patients with type 1 diabetes or type 2 diabetes have the following recommended glycemic goals:

- A$_{1c}$ less than 7.0%, less than 6.5%, or between 7% and 8%, depending on the specialty organization making such recommendations.
- Glucose management indicator via continuous glucose monitoring can be used as a replacement for A$_{1c}$, especially when A$_{1c}$ assessment might be inaccurate or difficult to obtain.
- Having glucose between 70 and 180 mg/dL more than 70% of the time.
- Having glucose less than 70 mg/dL less than 4% of the time.
- Having glucose less than 54 mg/dL less than 1% of the time.
- Having glucose greater than 180 mg/dL less than 25% of the time.
- Having glucose greater than 250 mg/dL less than 5% of the time.
- Having glycemic variability (% glycemic variability) $\leq 36\%$.

- Other goals may be recommended or considered:
  - Recommended goals are more stringent for pregnant patients with type 1 diabetes, pregnant patients with type 2 diabetes, and patients with gestational diabetes.
  - Recommended goals may be less stringent for patients with a history of or significant risk of hypoglycemia, hypoglycemia unawareness, other concurrent conditions, significantly compromised health status, limited life expectancy, or other circumstances that may make attaining more stringent glycemic goals unattainable or unsafe.

DISCLOSURES

- Research grants from:
  - National Institute of Nursing Research, National Institutes of Health
  - The Leona M. and Harry B. Helmsley Charitable Trust
- Educational grant from the American Academy of Family Physicians, via Abbott
- Advisory board and/or committee participation for:
  - American Diabetes Association
  - Association of Diabetes Care and Education Specialists
  - Cecelia Health
  - Dexcom
  - DiabetesWise
  - Jaeb Center for Health Research

REFERENCES

1. Clarke SF, Foster JR. A history of blood glucose meters and their role in self-monitoring of diabetes mellitus. Br J Biomed Sci 2012;69:83–93.
2. Guthrie DW, Humphreys S. Diabetes urine testing: an historical perspective. Diabetes Educator 1988;14(6):521–5.
3. Eknoyan G, Nagy J. A history of diabetes mellitus or how a disease of the kidneys evolved into a kidney disease. Adv Chronic Kidney Dis 2005;12(2):223–9.
4. Johnson G. Clinical lecture on the various modes of testing for sugar in the urine. Br Med J 1884;1(1201):1–4.
5. Hirsch IB, Battelino T, Peters AL, et al. Role of continuous glucose monitoring in diabetes treatment. Arlington, VA: American Diabetes Association; 2018.
6. Danne T, Nimri R, Battelino T, et al. International consensus on use of continuous glucose monitoring. Diabetes Care 2017;40(12):1631–40.
7. Harada Y, Harada K, Chin P Jr. Comparing self monitoring blood glucose devices and laboratory tests: over 25 years experience. Cureus 2019;11(12).
8. Ekhlaspour L, Mondesir D, Lautsch N, et al. Comparative accuracy of 17 point-of-care glucose meters. J Diabetes Sci Technology 2017;11(3):558–66.
9. Gifford R. Continuous glucose monitoring: 40 years, what we've learned and what's next. Chem Phys Chem 2013;14(10):2032–44.

10. Mastrototaro J, Shin J, Marcus A, et al, STAR 1 Clinical Trial Investigators. The accuracy and efficacy of real-time continuous glucose monitoring sensor in patients with type 1 diabetes. Diabetes Technology Ther 2008;10(5):385–90.

11. Garcia A, Rack-Gomer AL, Bhavaraju NC, et al. Dexcom G4AP: an advanced continuous glucose monitor for the artificial pancreas. J Diabetes Sci Technology 2013;7(6):1436–45.

12. Kropff J, Bruttomesso D, Doll W, et al. Accuracy of two continuous glucose monitoring systems: a head-to-head comparison under clinical research centre and daily life conditions. Diabetes Obes Metab 2015;17(4):343–9.

13. Chamberlain JJ. Continuous glucose monitoring systems: categories and features. Role of continuous glucose monitoring in diabetes treatment. Arlington, Virginia: American Diabetes Association; 2018.

14. Edelman SV, Argento NB, Pettus J, et al. Clinical implications of real-time and intermittently scanned continuous glucose monitoring. Diabetes Care 2018;41(11):2265–74.

15. Christiansen MP, Garg SK, Brazg R, et al. Accuracy of a fourth-generation subcutaneous continuous glucose sensor. Diabetes Technology Ther 2017;19(8):446–56.

16. Aronson R, Abitbol A, Tweden KS. First assessment of the performance of an implantable continuous glucose monitoring system through 180 days in a primarily adolescent population with type 1 diabetes. Diabetes Obes Metab 2019;21(7):1689–94.

17. Cowart K. Expanding flash continuous glucose monitoring technology to a broader population. Clin Diabetes 2021;cd200066.

18. Laiteerapong N, Ham SA, Gao Y, et al. The legacy effect in type 2 diabetes: impact of early glycemic control on future complications (The Diabetes & Aging Study). Diabetes Care 2019;42:416–26.

19. Stratton IM, Adler AI, Neil HAW, et al. Association of glycaemia with macrovascular and microvascular complications of type 2 diabetes (UKPDS 35): prospective observational study. BMJ 2000;321:405–12.

20. Little RR, Rohlfing CL, Sacks DB. National Glycohemoglobin Standardization Program (NGSP) Steering Committee. Status of hemoglobin A1c measurement and goals for improvement: from chaos to order for improving diabetes care. Clin Chem 2011;57:205–14.

21. Glycemic Targets: Standards of Medical care in diabetes–2021. Diabetes Care 2021;44(Suppl. 1):S73–84.

22. Radin MS. Pitfalls in hemoglobin A1c measurement: when results may be misleading. J Gen Intern Med 2014;29(2):388–94.

23. Imran SA, Agarwal G, Bajaj HS, et al. Targets for glycemic control. Can J Diabetes 2018;42:S42–6.

24. Qaseem A, Wilt TJ, Kansagara D, et al. Hemoglobin A1c targets for glycemic control with pharmacologic therapy for nonpregnant adults with type 2 diabetes mellitus: a guidance statement update from the American College of Physicians. Ann Intern Med 2018;168(8):569–76.

25. Garber AJ, Handelsman Y, Grunberger G, et al. Consensus statement by the American Association of Clinical Endocrinologists and American College of Endocrinology on the comprehensive type 2 diabetes management algorithm–2020 executive summary. Endocr Pract 2020;26(1):107–39.

26. Battelino T, Danne T, Bergenstal RM, et al. Clinical targets for continuous glucose monitoring data interpretation: recommendations from the international consensus on time in range. Diabetes Care 2019;42(8):1593–603.

Atypical Diabetes and Management Considerations

Shivajirao Prakash Patil, MD, MPH, BC-ADM, FAAFP*

KEYWORDS

- Atypical diabetes • Latent autoimmune diabetes in adults (LADA)
- Ketosis-prone diabetes mellitus (KPDM)

KEY POINTS

- Patients with latent autoimmune diabetes in adults (LADA) and ketosis-prone diabetes mellitus (KPDM) are commonly misdiagnosed as having type 1and type 2 diabetes mellitus, respectively.
- Evaluation of C-peptide levels along with use of specific risk scores based on clinical features helps evaluate for diabetes-specific autoantibody screening in adult patients at the onset of diabetes diagnosis to rule out LADA.
- Patients with LADA have the same diabetes-specific autoantibodies but slower progression toward an absolute insulin deficiency as compared with classical childhood-onset type 1 diabetes mellitus.
- Evaluation for KPDM includes checking diabetes-specific antibodies and C-peptide level at the close hospital follow-up appointment after the index diabetic ketoacidosis episode.
- After initial intensive insulin therapy, patients with KPDM maintain near-normoglycemia remission from insulin for many years.

BACKGROUND

Before 1936, when Sir Harold Percival Himsworth differentiated diabetes mellitus into "insulin-sensitive" and "insulin-insensitive" forms, diabetes mellitus was thought to be a uniform disease of insulin deficiency. Sir Himsworth found that several individuals with diabetes mellitus had insulin resistance instead of insulin deficiency.[1] The terms type 1 diabetes and type 2 diabetes were first used in 1951.[2] In 1979, the National Diabetes Data Group named types of diabetes mellitus based on their clinical presentation as "insulin-dependent diabetes mellitus" (IDDM) and "non-insulin-dependent diabetes mellitus" (NIDDM).[3] However, some patients did not fit into this classification system because of the discovery of other types of diabetes mellitus with specific pathophysiology, along with the evolution of other diabetes mellitus treatment options. In

Department of Family Medicine, Brody School of Medicine, East Carolina University, 101 Heart Drive, Mail Stop 654, Greenville, NC 278347, USA
* Corresponding Author.
E-mail address: patils@ecu.edu

Prim Care Clin Office Pract 49 (2022) 225–237
https://doi.org/10.1016/j.pop.2021.11.003
0095-4543/22/© 2021 Elsevier Inc. All rights reserved.

June 1997, an international committee of experts from the American Diabetes Association (ADA) and the World Health Organization released a report with a new classification of diabetes mellitus. This classification system identified four types of diabetes mellitus: type 1 diabetes mellitus (T1DM), type 2 diabetes mellitus (T2DM), "other specific types," and gestational diabetes.[4] Although the ADA continues to endorse this new classification system, it also recognizes that the type of diabetes mellitus is not always straightforward at presentation when misdiagnosis is common in all age groups and diagnosis becomes evident over time.[5] This article covers two such atypical types of diabetes mellitus, namely latent autoimmune diabetes of adults (LADA) and ketosis-prone diabetes mellitus (KPDM), both of which are at increased risk of misdiagnosis, resulting in suboptimal management. In the United States, primary care providers manage about 90% of patients with diabetes mellitus.[6] It is important to raise their awareness of these atypical types of diabetes mellitus. **Table 1** compares characteristics of T1DM, T2DM, LADA and KPDM.

LATENT AUTOIMMUNE DIABETES OF ADULTS
Introduction

LADA is a term used to describe a heterogenous form of autoimmune diabetes that resembles type 1 diabetes but has an onset during adulthood and slower progression toward an absolute insulin deficiency as compared with classical childhood-onset T1DM, which requires immediate exogenous insulin therapy.[7] About 2% to 12% of all patients with diabetes mellitus may have LADA, which likely contributes to a significant proportion of the increasing global prevalence of diabetes mellitus.[8] Most patients with LADA do not require insulin at diagnosis; however, they also have diabetes-specific autoantibodies (DAAs). Thus, they share features of both T1DM and T2DM and are at risk of being misdiagnosed as having T2DM.[9] It is important for clinicians to understand the slowly progressive autoimmune β-cell destruction in LADA,[10] which requires earlier insulin initiation before worsening of glycemic control or development of potentially life-threatening diabetic ketoacidosis (DKA).[11,12] Despite being a well-recognized form of diabetes mellitus, there have been uncertainties concerning almost all aspects of LADA, including diagnostic criteria, epidemiology, natural history, and pathogenesis, resulting in no clear strategies for its management[5,13] until an international expert panel released a consensus statement on management of LADA in 2020.[9]

Epidemiology

LADA may account for 2% to 12% of all cases of diabetes mellitus according to epidemiologic studies from North America, Europe, and Asia.[8,14–16] It is more prevalent in Caucasians than among African American, Hispanic, and Asian individuals.[15–17] Studies from China, Korea, India, and United Arab Emirates reported a prevalence of 5.7%, 4.4% to 5.3%, 2.6% to 3.2%, and 2.6%, respectively.[18–23] Thus, prevalence of LADA varies by geographic area and ethnicity.

Pathophysiology

Patients with LADA have the same DAAs as patients with childhood-onset classical T1DM. These DAAs are glutamic acid decarboxylase autoantibodies (GADA), insulin autoantibodies (IAA), protein tyrosine phosphatase IA-2 (IA-2A), and islet-specific zinc transporter isoform 8 autoantibodies (ZnT8). Although patients with LADA have at least one of these DAAs, they tend to have fewer multiple DAAs, unlike patients with T1DM. In addition, the autoimmune β-cell destruction in LADA is slower than

Table 1
Characteristics of different types of diabetes

	Type 1 Diabetes Mellitus	Type 2 Diabetes Mellitus	Latent Autoimmune Diabetes in Adults	Ketosis-Prone Diabetes Mellitus
Common age of presentation	Childhood, adolescence	Adolescence, adulthood	Adulthood (typically between 30 and 50 y)	Adolescence, adulthood
Ethnicity	Variable but predominantly Caucasian	Variable	Variable but predominantly Caucasian	Variable but predominantly African American
Symptoms at presentation	Acute; could be in DKA	Variable (none/subclinical/subacute/acute)	Acute or subclinical; rarely DKA	Acute, DKA
Body mass index	Normal	Overweight or obese	Normal or overweight	Overweight or obese
Diabetes-specific antibodies	Present	Absent	Present	Absent
C-peptide level at diagnosis	Low to undetectable	Normal to high (progressively decrease to low as disease advances)	Low to normal (progressively decrease to undetectable as disease advances)	Normal
Management	Insulin	ADA/EASD management algorithm for T2DM management	Guided by C-peptide level; typically initial insulin dependence followed by total insulin dependency within months to years. May use T2DM medications with or without insulin depending on C-peptide level. Avoid sulfonylureas and caution with SGLT-2 inhibitors	Insulin during initial acute phase, then lifestyle modifications. Similar to T2DM management if hyperglycemia is noted except avoid SGLT-2 inhibitors. Prompt insulin initiation for hyperglycemia and ketosis

Abbreviation: DKA, Diabetic ketoacidosis; ADA, American Diabetes Association; EASD, Europian Association for the Study of Diabetes; SGLT-2, Sodium–glucose cotransporter-2; T2DM, type 2 diabetes mellitus.
Data from Refs.[5,9,25,40,44,49]

that in T1DM, leading to a later onset of detectable hyperglycemia. The reason for this is not clearly understood: It is unclear if the β-cell damage is due to immune dysfunction itself or if DAAs are formed due to other pathogenic processes in genetically susceptible individuals.[17] Genome-wide association studies have demonstrated that LADA shares the genetic features of both T1DM and T2DM.[24] Two separate causative pathways of islet autoimmunity have been suggested. In the first pathway, specific immunologic triggers in leaner individuals with moderate T1DM genetic susceptibility lead to the development of GADA. The second causative pathway involves a low-grade chronic inflammatory process in obese individuals with T2DM genetic susceptibility, leading to the development of IA-2 antibodies.[25]

Diagnosis

Characterizing diagnostic criteria for LADA has been challenging, as it shares immunogenetic and phenotypic features of both T1DM and T2DM.[9] Various clinical features and laboratory markers have been used in different studies. The Immunology of Diabetes Society established 3 criteria to diagnose LADA: age at diagnosis of at least 30 years, presence of at least one of the 4 circulating DAAs, and having not been treated with insulin within the first 6 months after diagnosis.[8] However, each of these criteria has limitations, making the precise diagnosis of LADA challenging. Although different age cutoffs have been used in scientific literature, more than 30 years has been commonly used. Islet cell autoantibodies are not specific to LADA, as they are also present in T1DM, and insulin initiation depends on the degree of hyperglycemia and clinical presentation at diagnosis, provider judgment, and patient factors, such as willingness to take insulin, and cost.

A 5-point clinical screening tool has been proposed to identify adults with diabetes mellitus at higher risk for LADA. Presence of 2 or more out of 5 distinguishing clinical features (age of onset at <50 years, acute symptoms of hyperglycemia at onset, body mass index [BMI] <25 kg/m^2, personal history of autoimmune disease, or family history of autoimmune disease) at diagnosis of diabetes mellitus had 90% sensitivity and 71% specificity for detecting LADA, which should prompt testing for DAAs. The presence of one or none of these clinical features had a negative predictive value of 99%.[26]

A C-peptide level is used to guide LADA management right from the diagnosis. Hyperglycemia and hypoglycemia can affect C-peptide level, so C-peptide should always be measured in a nonacute stable situation with a concomitant blood glucose level, which should ideally be between 80 and 180 mg/dL. Although testing for DAAs is expensive and may not be available universally, C-peptide assays are relatively inexpensive and widely available.[9] Use of the clinical risk tool at the diagnosis of diabetes mellitus to identify individuals at higher risk of LADA and evaluation of C-peptide level should be considered before ordering DAAs. Patients with 2 or more clinical features should undergo DAAs testing. Patients with 1 clinical feature and low C-peptide level should also have DAAs testing. GADA is the most commonly occurring DAA in LADA,[9] so it should be checked first to limit the cost. If GADA is negative and there is still strong clinical suspicion of LADA, the other 3 DAAs should be ordered.[9,17,25]

Management

Heterogeneity among patients with LADA along with lack of good-quality, long-term randomized controlled trials makes it challenging to formulate its therapeutic plan. Patients with LADA have residual β-cell function at diagnosis, so the management goal is to preserve β-cell function while improving glycemic control.[9,17] The plan should be individualized depending on the patient's clinical features and laboratory data.

Lifestyle modifications are an important aspect of the management of all types of diabetes mellitus, although studies in LADA are limited. All patients with LADA should receive structured diabetes and diet education. Supervised weight loss treatment is indicated in patients with LADA and obesity along with assistance with smoking cessation in patients who smoke. Screening, prevention, and management of microvascular and macrovascular complications are important in patients with LADA, similar to all types of DM.[9]

Insulin has been shown to achieve effective and safe glycemic control in patients with LADA[27–29] and is essential in all patients with undetectable C-peptide. However, the time to initiate insulin therapy during early stages in patients with substantial residual β-cell function is not well studied.[9] Metformin has been shown to improve insulin sensitivity, resulting in the reduction of daily insulin requirement without long-term glycemic improvement, and to reduce weight, low-density lipoprotein cholesterol and atherosclerosis progression in patients with T1DM.[30,31] However, there is limited evidence to support or avoid its use in patients with LADA.[9] Although there are a few studies that showed thiazolidinediones (TZD) helped preserve β-cell function in patients with LADA,[32,33] more studies are needed to replicate this finding and justify its use, as TZDs have a significant side-effect profile, including weight gain and fluid retention. Thus, metformin and TZDs may be helpful in patients with LADA who have features of insulin resistance, but evidence of their efficacy is inconclusive, and more studies are needed.[9]

Although sulfonylureas are not recommended in patients with LADA owing to causing deterioration of β-cell function,[9,29,33,34] incretin-based therapies are gaining more attention lately for use in patients with residual β-cell function. A few studies have demonstrated that dipeptidyl peptidase 4 (DPP-4) inhibitors safely improved glycemic control in patients with LADA while preserving β-cell function.[34–36] Hence, DPP-4 inhibitors are emerging as a potential therapy for the management of LADA. GLP-1 receptor agonists (GLP-1 RAs) have been shown to improve glycemic control in patients with LADA and residual β-cell function.[37] Although more evidence is needed to further justify the use of these incretin-based therapies in LADA, these might be used as an add-on therapy to insulin to sustain residual β-cell function while achieving glycemic control.[9] Simultaneous use of a DPP-4 inhibitor and a GLP-1 RA is not recommended owing to lack of evidence on glycemic control and safety.[38] Although no studies have been conducted on sodium-glucose cotransporter-2 (SGLT-2) inhibitors in LADA, they may have a role in its management because of their growing evidence in the management of patients with T2DM and selected patients with T1DM.[39,40] However, their risk of ketoacidosis could be a concern, especially in patients with C-peptide levels ≤0.7 nmol/L.[39] One small study demonstrated the safety of immune intervention along with its beneficial effect on β-cell function in LADA, but more evidence is required before it can be recommended.[41]

A C-peptide level is used to guide the medication management right from the diagnosis of LADA, as mentioned above. If C-peptide levels are less than 0.3 nmol/L, then intensive insulin therapy (eg, multiple daily insulin injections, insulin pump) is recommended, similar to the recommendations for patients with T1DM. The ADA/European Association for the Study of Diabetes (EASD) algorithm for T2DM recommends metformin as the first-line medication along with lifestyle modifications, while considering factors, such as atherosclerotic cardiovascular disease, hear failure, chronic kidney disease, hypoglycemia risk, need for weight loss, and cost, to decide on additional agents.[9,40] A modified ADA/EASD algorithm for T2DM is suggested for patients with LADA with C-peptide levels greater than 0.7 nmol/L.[9] This modification includes avoiding sulfonylureas, as they have been shown to deteriorate β-cell function,[29,33,34] and careful use of SGLT-2 inhibitors, which increases the risk of ketoacidosis.[39] If a patient's blood glucose levels deteriorate, C-peptide level should be promptly repeated in these patients to assess the need for insulin.[9] C-peptide levels between 0.3 and 0.7 nmol/L fall into a "gray area," and the modified ADA/EASD algorithm for type 2 diabetes mentioned above is recommended. However, their combination with insulin should be considered for glycemic control and prevention of complications. Patients in this group should have C-peptide monitored at least every 6 months, and those with marked hyperglycemia may need to be started on insulin with frequent follow-up.[9]

CLINICS CARE POINTS

- Patients with latent autoimmune diabetes in adults constitute up to 12% of all patients with diabetes in clinic settings. Patients share immunogenic and phenotypic features of both type 2 diabetes and type 2 diabetes mellitus. They are often misdiagnosed as having type 2 diabetes mellitus, which increases the risk of delay in insulin initiation when hyperglycemia is noted.

- Use of the clinical risk tool (age of onset <50 years, acute symptoms of hyperglycemia at onset, body mass index <25 kg/m^2, personal history of autoimmune disease, or family history of autoimmune disease) at the diagnosis of diabetes mellitus and evaluation of C-peptide level help identify individuals at higher risk of latent autoimmune diabetes in adults before ordering diabetes-specific autoantibodies.

- Management of latent autoimmune diabetes in adults requires a careful personalized strategy. C-peptide level should be monitored every 6 months to guide treatment. Patients with low C-peptide levels should be started on insulin.

- Noninsulin agents may be used with or without insulin in patients with residual β-cell function based on a C-peptide level. Insulin sensitizers (metformin and thiazolidinediones) may be used in patients with evidence of insulin resistance. DPP4-inhibitors and GLP-1 receptor agonists help preserve β-cell function while achieving glycemic control. SGLT-2 inhibitors should be used carefully because of their risk of ketosis. Sulfonylureas should be avoided, as they deteriorate β-cell function.

KETOSIS-PRONE DIABETES MELLITUS
Introduction

DKA is a life-threatening but preventable complication of diabetes mellitus characterized by hyperglycemia, metabolic acidosis, and ketonemia resulting from an absolute or relative insulin deficiency.[42] DKA hospitalizations are expensive and are increasing in the United States.[43] DKA was previously thought to occur almost exclusively in patients with T1DM.[44] However, over the last few decades, DKA has been noted to occur at presentation in patients without classic features of autoimmune T1DM.[45–62] This condition is called "ketosis-prone diabetes mellitus" (KPDM).[63]

Epidemiology

In the 1960s, a few adult patients with DKA in West Africa were able to discontinue insulin therapy after a relatively short time and remained in near-normoglycemia for several months to years. This condition was named "temporary diabetes" in adult Nigerians.[45,46] Further reports from other African groups noted challenges in classifying similar patients as having either T1DM or T2DM at the time of their initial presentation. In 1987, a small group of young African American patients who presented with severe hyperglycemia or DKA was noted to have clinical and metabolic features of

T2DM. They called it "atypical diabetes."[47] In the 1990s, a group of black patients of Caribbean and African origin presented with DKA. They did not have DAAs, and most of them were able to discontinue insulin after initial brief intensive insulin therapy.[48–50] It was referred to as "Flatbush diabetes."[48] Since then, similar cases have been reported in Native American, Japanese, Chinese, Asian Indian, Pakistani, Korean, Thai, Hispanic, Peruvian, and Caucasian (US and European) populations.[51–62] Although the exact prevalence of KPDM is unknown, there is a higher prevalence in men compared with women.[63]

Pathophysiology

KPDM is characterized by an initial episode of DKA in a patient without classic features of T1DM. Although several studies demonstrated initial decompensation of -cell function and subsequent recovery, their cause is unknown, and the reason for predisposition toward ketosis is not clearly understood. Autoimmune, viral (eg, human herpes virus 8), and genetic (eg, glucose-6-phosphate dehydrogenase i.e. G6PD deficiency) causes have been examined along with metabolic derangements, such as glucotoxicity and lipotoxicity.[64–66] However, some of these findings could not be confirmed on follow-up studies or studies in different cohorts of patients with KPDM.[64]

Classification

The goal of classifying patients who present with new-onset DKA is to help clinicians predict which patients require transient versus long-term insulin therapy. In 2003, the Aß system was introduced to differentiate such patients into 4 subgroups depending on the presence or absence of DAAs (indicated as "A") and the presence or absence of pancreatic ß-cell functional reserve (indicated as "ß") measured by a fasting C-peptide level greater than 1 ng/mL or stimulated C-peptide level $\geq$1.5 ng/mL in a stable state after the index DKA episode. The 4 subgroups are A+ß− (DAAs present and ß-cell function absent), A+ß+ (DAAs and ß-cell function present), A−ß+ (DAAs absent and ß-cell function absent), and A−ß− (DAAs and ß-cell function absent).[67] This Aß classification system has a sensitivity of 99.4% and specificity of 95.9%.[68] Patients with KPDM (A−ß+ status) follow a clinical course that includes ß-cell recovery with initial intensive insulin therapy and maintain near-normoglycemia remission from insulin for many years. Patients with T1DM (A+ß− status) require lifelong insulin therapy.[65]

Management

Patients with KPDM typically present in DKA with acute and very recent history (usually <4 weeks) of hyperglycemic symptoms, such as polyuria, polydipsia, and weight loss.[49,64] Presentation of DKA is usually very similar to DKA in T1DM, including severe hyperglycemia greater than 500 mg/dL, hemoglobin A1c (HbA$_{1c}$) greater than 10%, and a blood pH less than 7.30 along with ketoacidosis.[49,53,55] Most patients with KPDM have phenotypical characteristic of T2DM, such as acanthosis nigricans, obesity, abdominal adiposity,[49] and a strong family history of T2DM.[69] Management of DKA in KPDM is the same as DKA management in T1DM; however, unlike patients with T1DM, patients with KPDM often require a relatively higher subcutaneous starting insulin dose of 0.8 to 1.2 units/kg per day owing to insulin resistance.[49,64] After 2 to 12 weeks, insulin requirement usually decreases, and about 70% of patients achieve near-normoglycemic remission.[67,70] Umpierrez and colleagues[49] defined near-normoglycemia remission as HbA$_{1c}$ less than 7% and the ability to maintain fasting blood glucose less than 130 mg/dL off subcutaneous insulin therapy for at least

1 week, whereas others have defined near-normoglycemia remission differently.[71] The period of remission varies from 6 to 120 months.[67]

After discharge, patients should remain on insulin therapy until they are followed up in the clinic within 1 to 3 weeks to allow for glucotoxicity resolution. During this visit, DAAs (GADA, IAA, IA-2, and if available, ZnT8 antibodies) and β-cell secretory reserve should be performed to classify patients appropriately according to the Aβ system, which helps predict clinical course and evaluate for insulin therapy. β-cell secretory reserve is measured by a fasting or stimulated C-peptide level as described above. It is the strongest predictor of long-term glycemic control and insulin dependence.[44] Once classified as having KPDM (A−β+ status), insulin weaning protocol is started depending on glycemic control and lifestyle factors, such as diet and exercise. If fasting and bedtime blood glucose values are consistently less than 130 mg/dL and less than 180 mg/dL, respectively, total daily insulin dose should be reduced by 50%. Patients should continue self-monitoring of blood glucose and maintain close follow-up with their clinic provider to continue insulin weaning protocol.

After discontinuation of insulin therapy, if home blood glucose values remain at goal, continue with lifestyle modification and monitor without pharmacologic therapy. If blood glucose values increase without the development of ketosis, start noninsulin T2DM agents. Metformin,[70] DPP4-inhibitors,[70] GLP-1 Ras,[72] and sulfonylurea[73,74] have been studied to be efficacious in prolonging near-normoglycemia. Sulfonylureas, however, increase the risk of hypoglycemia and weight gain. As patients with KPDM tend to develop DKA, SGLT-2 inhibitors should be avoided because of the risk of euglycemic ketosis.[44] Despite lifestyle modification and effective medication management, patients with KPDM are at risk of hyperglycemia and DKA. Patients should be educated to seek immediate medical attention when persistent hyperglycemia is noted. Checking for significant ketosis if the blood glucose level increases to greater than 200 mg/dL is recommended.[44]

Screening and management of microvascular and macrovascular complications are important in patients with KPDM along with other standards of diabetes care for long-term management. This includes periodic counseling from a registered dietician and diabetes educator, physical activity for at least 150 minutes per week, weight loss, and smoking cessation if indicated.[44]

CLINICS CARE POINTS

- If ketosis-prone diabetes mellitus is incorrectly diagnosed as type 1 diabetes at presentation, the diagnosis may never subsequently be questioned, which may lead to unnecessary long-term insulin treatment with potential weight gain, hypoglycemia, implications for quality of life and employment, and health care cost.

- Patients with ketosis-prone diabetes mellitus need more careful education and follow-up than those with typical type 2 diabetes.

- Correct recognition of ketosis-prone diabetes mellitus by checking diabetes-specific autoantibodies and C-peptide levels at the close hospital follow-up appointment after the index DKA episode helps safe weaning of insulin over a period of months.

- Most patients can be treated successfully with lifestyle modifications unless hyperglycemia is noted, in which case noninsulin agents can be used (with the exception of SGLT-2 inhibitors).

- Patient education should focus on home blood glucose monitoring, allowing for appropriate early management of hyperglycemia and avoidance of diabetic ketoacidosis.

DISCLOSURE

The author has nothing to disclose.

REFERENCES

1. Kim SH. Measurement of insulin action: a tribute to Sir Harold Himsworth. Diabet Med 2011;28(12):1487–93.
2. Gale EA. The discovery of type 1 diabetes. Diabetes 2001;50(2):217–26.
3. Classification and diagnosis of diabetes mellitus and other categories of glucose intolerance. National Diabetes Data Group. Diabetes 1979;28(12):1039–57.
4. Report of the Expert Committee on the Diagnosis and Classification of Diabetes Mellitus. Diabetes Care Jul 1997;20(7):1183–97.
5. American Diabetes Association. 2. Classification and diagnosis of diabetes: standards of medical care in diabetes-2021. Diabetes Care 2021;44(Suppl 1):S15–33.
6. Davidson JA. The increasing role of primary care physicians in caring for patients with type 2 diabetes mellitus. Mayo Clin Proc 2010;85(12 Suppl):S3–4.
7. Guglielmi C, Palermo A, Pozzilli P. Latent autoimmune diabetes in the adults (LADA) in Asia: from pathogenesis and epidemiology to therapy. Diabetes Metab Res Rev 2012;28(Suppl 2):40–6.
8. Naik RG, Brooks-Worrell BM, Palmer JP. Latent autoimmune diabetes in adults. J Clin Endocrinol Metab 2009;94(12):4635–44.
9. Buzzetti R, Tuomi T, Mauricio D, et al. Management of latent autoimmune diabetes in adults: a consensus statement from an international expert panel. Diabetes 2020;69(10):2037–47.
10. Zhu Y, Qian L, Liu Q, et al. Glutamic acid decarboxylase autoantibody detection by electrochemiluminescence assay identifies latent autoimmune diabetes in adults with poor islet function. Diabetes Metab J 2020;44(2):260–6.
11. Thomas NJ, Lynam AL, Hill AV, et al. Type 1 diabetes defined by severe insulin deficiency occurs after 30 years of age and is commonly treated as type 2 diabetes. Diabetologia 2019;62(7):1167–72.
12. Lynam A, McDonald T, Hill A, et al. Development and validation of multivariable clinical diagnostic models to identify type 1 diabetes requiring rapid insulin therapy in adults aged 18-50 years. BMJ Open 2019;9(9):e031586.
13. Cernea S, Buzzetti R, Pozzilli P. Beta-cell protection and therapy for latent autoimmune diabetes in adults. Diabetes Care 2009;32(Suppl 2):S246–52.
14. Zinman B, Kahn SE, Haffner SM, et al. ADOPT Study Group. Phenotypic characteristics of GAD antibody-positive recently diagnosed patients with type 2 diabetes in North America and Europe. Diabetes 2004;53(12):3193–200.
15. Hawa MI, Kolb H, Schloot N, et al. Action LADA consortium. Adult-onset autoimmune diabetes in Europe is prevalent with a broad clinical phenotype: Action LADA 7. Diabetes Care 2013;36(4):908–13.
16. Zhou Z, Xiang Y, Ji L, et al. LADA China Study Group. Frequency, immunogenetics, and clinical characteristics of latent autoimmune diabetes in China (LADA China study): a nationwide, multicenter, clinic-based cross-sectional study. Diabetes 2013;62(2):543–50.
17. Pieralice S, Pozzilli P. Latent autoimmune diabetes in adults: a review on clinical implications and management. Diabetes Metab J 2018;42(6):451–64. https://doi.org/10.4093/dmj.2018.0190.

18. Qi X, Sun J, Wang J, et al. Prevalence and correlates of latent autoimmune diabetes in adults in Tianjin, China: a population-based cross-sectional study. Diabetes Care 2011;34(1):66–70.
19. Park Y, Hong S, Park L, et al. KNDP Collaboratory Group. LADA prevalence estimation and insulin dependency during follow-up. Diabetes Metab Res Rev 2011; 27(8):975–9.
20. Roh MO, Jung CH, Kim BY, et al. The prevalence and characteristics of latent autoimmune diabetes in adults (LADA) and its relation with chronic complications in a clinical department of a university hospital in Korea. Acta Diabetol 2013; 50(2):129–34.
21. Britten AC, Jones K, Törn C, et al. Latent autoimmune diabetes in adults in a South Asian population of the U.K. Diabetes Care 2007;30(12):3088–90.
22. Sachan A, Zaidi G, Sahu RP, et al. Low prevalence of latent autoimmune diabetes in adults in northern India. Diabet Med 2015;32(6):810–3.
23. Maddaloni E, Lessan N, Al Tikriti A, et al. Latent autoimmune diabetes in adults in the United Arab Emirates: clinical features and factors related to insulin-requirement. PLoS One 2015;10(8):e0131837.
24. Haller K, Kisand K, Pisarev H, et al. Insulin gene VNTR, CTLA-4 +49A/G and HLA-DQB1 alleles distinguish latent autoimmune diabetes in adults from type 1 diabetes and from type 2 diabetes group. Tissue Antigens 2007;69(2):121–7.
25. Buzzetti R, Zampetti S, Maddaloni E. Adult-onset autoimmune diabetes: current knowledge and implications for management. Nat Rev Endocrinol 2017;13(11): 674–86.
26. Fourlanos S, Perry C, Stein MS, et al. A clinical screening tool identifies autoimmune diabetes in adults. Diabetes Care 2006;29(5):970–5.
27. Thunander M, Thorgeirsson H, Törn C, et al. β-cell function and metabolic control in latent autoimmune diabetes in adults with early insulin versus conventional treatment: a 3-year follow-up. Eur J Endocrinol 2011;164(2):239–45.
28. Kobayashi T, Nakanishi K, Murase T, et al. Small doses of subcutaneous insulin as a strategy for preventing slowly progressive beta-cell failure in islet cell antibody-positive patients with clinical features of NIDDM. Diabetes 1996;45(5):622–6.
29. Maruyama T, Tanaka S, Shimada A, et al. Insulin intervention in slowly progressive insulin-dependent (type 1) diabetes mellitus. J Clin Endocrinol Metab 2008;93(6): 2115–21.
30. Cree-Green M, Bergman BC, Cengiz E, et al. Metformin improves peripheral insulin sensitivity in youth with type 1 diabetes. J Clin Endocrinol Metab 2019; 104(8):3265–78.
31. Livingstone R, Boyle JG, Petrie JR, REMOVAL Study Team. A new perspective on metformin therapy in type 1 diabetes. Diabetologia 2017;60(9):1594–600.
32. Zhou Z, Li X, Huang G, et al. Rosiglitazone combined with insulin preserves islet beta cell function in adult-onset latent autoimmune diabetes (LADA). Diabetes Metab Res Rev 2005;21(2):203–8.
33. Yang Z, Zhou Z, Li X, et al. Rosiglitazone preserves islet beta-cell function of adult-onset latent autoimmune diabetes in 3 years follow-up study. Diabetes Res Clin Pract 2009;83(1):54–60.
34. Johansen OE, Boehm BO, Grill V, et al. C-peptide levels in latent autoimmune diabetes in adults treated with linagliptin versus glimepiride: exploratory results from a 2-year double-blind, randomized, controlled study. Diabetes Care 2014;37(1): e11–2.

35. Zhao Y, Yang L, Xiang Y, et al. Dipeptidyl peptidase 4 inhibitor sitagliptin maintains β-cell function in patients with recent-onset latent autoimmune diabetes in adults: one year prospective study. J Clin Endocrinol Metab 2014;99(5):E876–80.
36. Awata T, Shimada A, Maruyama T, et al. Possible long-term efficacy of sitagliptin, a dipeptidyl peptidase-4 inhibitor, for slowly progressive type 1 diabetes (SPIDDM) in the stage of non-insulin-dependency: an open-label randomized controlled pilot trial (SPAN-S). Diabetes Ther 2017;8:1123–34.
37. Pozzilli P, Leslie RD, Peters AL, et al. Dulaglutide treatment results in effective glycaemic control in latent autoimmune diabetes in adults (LADA): a post-hoc analysis of the AWARD-2, -4 and -5 Trials. Diabetes Obes Metab 2018;20:1490–8.
38. Lajthia E, Bucheit JD, Nadpara PA, et al. Combination therapy with once-weekly glucagon like peptide-1 receptor agonists and dipeptidyl peptidase-4 inhibitors in type 2 diabetes: a case series. Pharm Pract (Granada) 2019;17(4):1588.
39. Danne T, Garg S, Peters AL, et al. International consensus on risk management of diabetic ketoacidosis in patients with type 1 diabetes treated with sodium-glucose cotransporter (SGLT) inhibitors. Diabetes Care 2019;42(6):1147–54.
40. American Diabetes Association. 9. Pharmacologic approaches to glycemic treatment: standards of medical care in diabetes - 2021. Diabetes Care 2021;44(Suppl. 1):S111–24.
41. Agardh CD, Lynch KF, Palmér M, et al. GAD65 vaccination: 5 years of follow-up in a randomized dose-escalating study in adult-onset autoimmune diabetes. Diabetologia 2009;1363–8.
42. Nyenwe EA, Kitabchi AE. The evolution of diabetic ketoacidosis: an update of its etiology, pathogenesis and management. Metabolism 2016;65(4):507–21.
43. Benoit SR, Zhang Y, Geiss LS, et al. Trends in diabetic ketoacidosis hospitalizations and in-hospital mortality — United States, 2000–2014. MMWR Morb Mortal Wkly Rep 2018;67:362–5.
44. Gaba R, Mehta P, Balasubramanyam A. Evaluation and management of ketosis-prone diabetes. Expert Rev Endocrinol Metab 2019;14(1):43–8.
45. Dodu SR. Diabetes in the tropics. Br Med J 1967;2(5554):747–50.
46. Adadevoh BK. "Temporary diabetes" in adult Nigerians. Trans R Soc Trop Med Hyg 1968;62(4):528–30.
47. Winter WE, Maclaren NK, Riley WJ, et al. Maturity-onset diabetes of youth in black Americans. N Engl J Med 1987;316(6):285–91.
48. Banerji MA, Chaiken RL, Huey H, et al. GAD antibody negative NIDDM in adult black subjects with diabetic ketoacidosis and increased frequency of human leukocyte antigen DR3 and DR4. Flatbush diabetes. Diabetes 1994;43(6):741–5.
49. Umpierrez GE, Casals MM, Gebhart SP, et al. Diabetic ketoacidosis in obese African-Americans. Diabetes 1995;44(7):790–5.
50. Umpierrez GE, Woo W, Hagopian WA, et al. Immunogenetic analysis suggests different pathogenesis for obese and lean African-Americans with diabetic ketoacidosis. Diabetes Care 1999;22(9):1517–23.
51. Aizawa T, Katakura M, Taguchi N, et al. Ketoacidosis-onset noninsulin dependent diabetes in Japanese subjects. Am J Med Sci 1995;310(5):198–201.
52. Wilson C, Krakoff J, Gohdes D. Ketoacidosis in Apache Indians with non-insulin-dependent diabetes mellitus. Arch Intern Med 1997;157(18):2098–100.
53. Balasubramanyam A, Zern JW, Hyman DJ, et al. New profiles of diabetic ketoacidosis: type 1 vs type 2 diabetes and the effect of ethnicity. Arch Intern Med 1999;159(19):2317–22.
54. Westphal SA. The occurrence of diabetic ketoacidosis in non-insulin-dependent diabetes and newly diagnosed diabetic adults. Am J Med 1996;101(1):19–24.

55. Pinero-Pilona A, Litonjua P, Aviles-Santa L, et al. Idiopathic type 1 diabetes in Dallas, Texas: a 5-year experience. Diabetes Care 2001;24(6):1014–8.

56. Pinto ME, Villena JE, Villena AE. Diabetic ketoacidosis in Peruvian patients with type 2 diabetes mellitus. Endocr Pract 2008;14(4):442–6.

57. Pitteloud N, Philippe J. Characteristics of Caucasian type 2 diabetic patients during ketoacidosis and at follow-up. Schweiz Med Wochenschr 2000;130(16):576–82.

58. Jabbar A, Farooqui K, Habib A, et al. Clinical characteristics and outcomes of diabetic ketoacidosis in Pakistani adults with type 2 diabetes mellitus. Diabet Med 2004;21(8):920–3.

59. Gupta RD, Ramachandran R, Gangadhara P, et al. Clinical characteristics, beta-cell dysfunction and treatment outcomes in patients with A−β+ ketosis-prone diabetes (KPD): the first identified cohort amongst Asian Indians. J Diabet Complications 2017;31(9):1401–7.

60. Tan KC, Mackay IR, Zimmet PZ, et al. Metabolic and immunologic features of Chinese patients with atypical diabetes mellitus. Diabetes Care 2000;23(3):335–8.

61. Kim MK, Lee SH, Kim JH, et al. Clinical characteristics of Korean patients with new-onset diabetes presenting with diabetic ketoacidosis. Diabetes Res Clin Pract 2009;85(1):e8–11.

62. Gupta P, Liu Y, Lapointe M, et al. Changes in circulating adiponectin, leptin, glucose and C-peptide in patients with ketosis-prone diabetes. Diabet Med 2015;32(5):692–700.

63. Kitabchi AE. Ketosis-prone diabetes–a new subgroup of patients with atypical type 1 and type 2 diabetes? J Clin Endocrinol Metab 2003;88(11):5087–9.

64. Vellanki P, Umpierrez GE. Diabetic ketoacidosis: a common debut of diabetes among African Americans with type 2 diabetes. Endocr Pract 2017;23(8):971–8.

65. Smiley D, Chandra P, Umpierrez GE. Update on diagnosis, pathogenesis and management of ketosis-prone type 2 diabetes mellitus. Diabetes Manag (Lond) 2011;1(6):589–600.

66. Pinero-Pilona A, Raskin P. Idiopathic type 1 diabetes. J Diabetes Complications 2001;15(6):328–35.

67. Mauvais-Jarvis F, Sobngwi E, Porcher R, et al. Ketosis-prone type 2 diabetes in patients of sub-Saharan African origin: clinical pathophysiology and natural history of beta-cell dysfunction and insulin resistance. Diabetes 2004;53(3):645–53.

68. Maldonado M, Hampe CS, Gaur LK, et al. Ketosis-prone diabetes: dissection of a heterogeneous syndrome using an immunogenetic and beta-cell functional classification, prospective analysis, and clinical outcomes. J Clin Endocrinol Metab 2003;88(11):5090–8.

69. Balasubramanyam A, Garza G, Rodriguez L, et al. Accuracy and predictive value of classification schemes for ketosis-prone diabetes. Diabetes Care 2006;29(12):2575–9.

70. Vellanki P, Smiley DD, Stefanovski D, et al. Randomized controlled study of metformin and sitagliptin on long-term normoglycemia remission in African American patients with hyperglycemic crises. Diabetes Care 2016;39(11):1948–55.

71. McFarlane SI, Chaiken RL, Hirsch S, et al. Near-normoglycaemic remission in African-Americans with type 2 diabetes mellitus is associated with recovery of beta cell function. Diabet Med 2001;18(1):10–6.

72. Retnakaran R, Kramer CK, Choi H, et al. Liraglutide and the preservation of pancreatic β-cell function in early type 2 diabetes: the LIBRA trial. Diabetes Care 2014;37(12):3270–8.

73. Umpierrez GE, Clark WS, Steen MT. Sulfonylurea treatment prevents recurrence of hyperglycemia in obese African-American patients with a history of hyperglycemic crises. Diabetes Care 1997;20(4):479–83.
74. Banerji MA, Chaiken RL, Lebovitz HE. Prolongation of near-normoglycemic remission in black NIDDM subjects with chronic low-dose sulfonylurea treatment. Diabetes 1995;44(4):466–70.

Diabetes-Related Microvascular Complications – A Practical Approach

Basem M. Mishriky, MD[a],*, Doyle M. Cummings, PharmD, FCP, FCCP[b],
James R. Powell, MD[a]

KEYWORDS

- Microvascular complications • Diabetic symmetric polyneuropathy
- Diabetic kidney disease • Diabetic retinopathy • Practical approach

KEY POINTS

- Screen for microvascular complications at the time of diagnosis of type 2 diabetes.
- Inspection of the feet is encouraged at every visit.
- Renal evaluation should be performed at least annually to screen for diabetic kidney disease.
- Retinal evaluation by an expert should be performed regularly.

DIABETIC SYMMETRIC POLYNEUROPATHY
What is Diabetic Symmetric Polyneuropathy?

Diabetic neuropathy is classified into diffuse neuropathy, mononeuropathy, and radi-culopathy/polyradiculopathy.[1] Diabetic symmetric polyneuropathy (DSPN) is the most common form of diffuse neuropathy, which is the most common form of diabetic neuropathy.[1] DSPN affects 50% of individuals with type 2 diabetes (T2DM) after 10 years of disease duration and at least 20% of individuals with type 1 diabetes (T1DM) after 20 years of diagnosis.[1] DSPN can be referred to as distal symmetric polyneuropathy or even, although less accurate, as diabetic neuropathy.[2]

The American Academy of Neurology, the American Association of Electrodiagnostic Medicine, and the American Academy of Physical Medicine and Rehabilitation define distal symmetric polyneuropathy (including DSPN) as polyneuropathy that must begin in the feet and include symptoms and signs that are the same on both sides of the body.[3,4] The symptoms may be primarily sensory, primarily motor, or combined. The

[a] Department of Internal Medicine, East Carolina University, 521 Moye Boulevard, 2nd Floor, Greenville, NC 27834, USA; [b] Department of Family Medicine, East Carolina University, 101 Heart Drive, Greenville, NC 27834, USA
* Corresponding author.
E-mail address: mishrikyb@ecu.edu

Prim Care Clin Office Pract 49 (2022) 239–254
https://doi.org/10.1016/j.pop.2021.11.008
0095-4543/22/© 2021 Elsevier Inc. All rights reserved.
primarycare.theclinics.com

signs may include pain, impairment to touch, impairment to proprioception, weakness and atrophy of muscles, depressed/absent ankle reflexes, or autonomic system.[3,4] Signs are better predictors of polyneuropathy compared with symptoms and multiple concurrent abnormalities provide greater sensitivity in predicting polyneuropathy.

In the position statement by the American Diabetes Association (ADA), DSPN is defined as the presence of symptoms or signs of peripheral nerve dysfunctions after excluding other causes.[1]

Can Patients without Numbness, Tingling, or Pain in the Feet have Diabetic Symmetric Polyneuropathy, and Why is this Important?

Around 50% of individuals with DSPN are asymptomatic; therefore, the absence of symptoms cannot rule out DSPN.[1] As DSPN with or without deformity increases the risk of amputation,[5] diabetic foot examinations are extremely important to allow the early identification of DSPN to prevent progression to ulcerations and amputations.

How do Individuals with Diabetic Symmetric Polyneuropathy Present?

The clinical presentation can be classified according to the type of nerve affected (motor, sensory, or autonomic) or according to the size of nerve fiber involvement (either small-fiber or large-fiber involvement) (**Fig. 1**).

A simplified view of the PNS

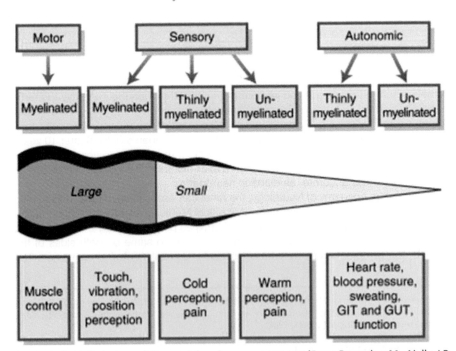

Fig. 1. A simplified view of the peripheral nervous system. (*From* Brownlee M, Aiello LP, Cooper ME, Vinik AI, Plutzky J, and Boulton AJM. Chapter 33: Complications of diabetes mellitus. In: Kronenberg HM, Larsen PR, Melmed S, and Polonsky KS, eds. Williams Textbook of Endocrinology. 13th ed. Elsevier: 2016: 1484-1581; with permission.)

Small-fiber involvement

Small-fibers usually involve sensory and autonomic nerves. The most common and early symptom is neuropathic pain which is characterized by burning, lancinating, and shooting pain that worsens at night. It may be associated with an unpleasant sensation of burning (dysesthesias), an exaggerated response to painful stimuli (hyperalgesia), and/or an exaggerated pain evoked by contact with socks, shoes, or bedclothes (allodynia).[1,5] Defects in the autonomic function of the nerves may result in decreased sweating, dry skin, impaired vasomotor function, and cold feet.[5,6]

Large-fiber involvement

Large-fibers usually involve sensory and/or motor nerves. Following the small-fiber involvement, the normal progression of symptoms is to develop numbness, tingling, and loss of protective sensations.[1,5,6] This is accompanied by loss of position sense and loss of reflexes. Later, muscle wasting with subsequent foot deformities develops.[5]

While the onset of symptoms is usually insidious, some patients may have an acute onset of symptoms.[5] DSPN typically affects the lower extremities in a stocking-like distribution. In more severe cases and by the time the symptoms reach the knees, the hands may be involved. While initially it may be reversible, the disappearance of pain in later stages should be interpreted as nerve death and is a worrisome sign.[6]

Is Ongoing Foot Pain and Numbness in Individuals with Diabetes Always Diabetic Symmetric Polyneuropathy?

While DSPN is principally a clinical diagnosis, health care providers (HCP) need to ensure that other causes of neuropathy are ruled out. A reasonable initial workup may include[1]:

- Complete blood count
- Basic metabolic panel
- Thyroid-stimulating hormone
- Serum vitamin B12 and folic acid levels
- HIV, if the patient is at high risk
- Serum protein electrophoresis to evaluate multiple myeloma if clinically suspected

While the confirmation of pathologic diagnosis may require nerve conduction studies and a biopsy, they are rarely needed in clinical practice.

What are the Criteria for Requesting a Nerve Conduction Study (Possible Reasons for Specialist Referral)?

- Patients with asymmetric symptoms[6]
- Rapid development or progression[6]
- Progression of symptoms despite adequate glycemic control[6]
- Symptoms more common in the hands[6]

It should be noted that if suspicion is high, but the nerve conduction studies are negative, a skin biopsy may still be needed to evaluate for small-fiber disease.[3]

What are the Minimum Criteria Required to Diagnose Diabetic Symmetric Polyneuropathy?

The Toronto Consensus has defined the minimal criteria for the diagnosis of DSPN[5]:

- Possible DSPN: The presence of a symptom or sign of DSPN.
- Probable DSPN: The presence of a combination of symptoms and signs.

- Confirmed DSPN: The presence of a symptom or sign confirmed with an abnormal nerve conduction study.

When Should the Health Care Providers Screen for Diabetic Symmetric Polyneuropathy?

While individuals with T1DM should be screened after 5 years from diagnosis, individuals with T2DM should be screened at the time of diagnosis as T2DM duration before diagnosis may not be known. While guidelines recommend screening for DSPN by examining the feet at least once yearly, it is our practice to examine/inspect the patient's feet at every visit. This practice of examining the feet at every visit reinforces the importance of the patient checking their own feet daily.

How Should the Health Care Providers Screen for Diabetic Symmetric Polyneuropathy?

History

The patient should be asked about symptoms of DSPN (including burning/shooting pain, numbness, tingling, coldness of the feet) at every visit. The history should also include symptoms of claudication, rest pain, and/or nonhealing ulcer. Past history should address any prior ulceration, amputation, Charcot joint, or vascular surgery. Finally, smoking history should be obtained.

Examination

A careful inspection of the feet in a well-lit room should always be carried out after the patient has removed their shoes and socks.

The foot examination should include[7]:

Inspection for:

- Dryness or cracking, infection, and calluses/corns of the skin.
- Evidence of deformities (eg, claw toes, hammer toes, overlapping toes, bunion).
- Evidence of muscle wasting.

Neurologic assessment:

This requires testing for sensation: usually, a monofilament test combined with one or more tests for both large-fiber involvement (such as vibration sense, reflexes, proprioception) and small-fiber involvement (such as pinprick sensation and thermal discrimination).

- Testing for protective sensations (large-nerve fiber): It is recommended to use at least a 5.07 (10-g) monofilament to screen for loss of protective sensations. While screening for the loss of protective sensations using the 5.07 (10-g) monofilament may be convenient during a busy clinical practice,[8] it is advised to follow clinical progression by using a graded monofilament kit with different target forces.[9–11] Individuals with diabetes but no DSPN should be able to sense the 4.31 (2-g) and the 3.61 (0.4-g) monofilaments.[9–11] It is reasonable to start with the 3.61 (0.4-g) monofilament and proceed in order of increasing stiffness.[9]

Steps to perform the monofilament testing:
- Explain the test to the patient before starting.
- The sensation of pressure with the monofilament should first be demonstrated to the patient on a proximal site, usually the hands. The patient should be instructed to report if a touch is felt, then specify the site they felt the touch.
- The patient should close their eyes while being tested.
- Areas of callus, abrasion, or scarring should be avoided.
- The monofilament is pressed perpendicular to the skin for approximately 1 second while it is buckling to ensure that the target force is delivered to the tested site.

- ○ At least 4 sites should be tested on each foot (plantar surface of the big toe, 1st, 3rd, and 5th metatarsal heads). If using ≤4.08 (1-g) monofilament, the stimulus can be applied up to 3 times to elicit a response. If using greater than 4.08 (1-g) monofilament, the stimulus should be applied only once.
- ○ If a graded monofilament kit is available, the examiner may begin with a 3.61 (0.4-g) monofilament. If the patient does not respond to the stimulus, choose the next largest monofilament. If a graded monofilament kit is not available, screening with a 5.07 (10-g) monofilament should be used.
- ○ A test is considered abnormal if sensation is lost at one or more of the tested sites.[7]

If a 5.07 (10-g) monofilament is not available, an Ipswich touch test may be used instead.[12] This is a simple, cheap, and equally sensitive and specific test when compared with monofilament testing.[12] The patient should close their eyes and the examiner should rest an index finger (like a feather touching the skin) on the tip of the 1st, 3rd, and 5th toes of both feet. This should last for one to 2 seconds. The patients should indicate if they feel the touch. A test is considered abnormal if the patient cannot feel any 2 examined sites.

- • Testing for vibratory sensations (large-nerve fiber): This should be done using a 128-Hz tuning fork.

Steps to perform the tuning fork testing:
- ○ Explain the test to the patient before starting.
- ○ The vibration sense should first be demonstrated to the patient usually over the thumb. The patient should be made aware that it is the sensation of vibration, not the pressure, that is being tested.
- ○ The vibrating tuning fork should be placed over the tip of the big toe or at the base of the great toenail (or at the medial malleolus if there is toe amputation[13]) bilaterally for at least 8 to 10 seconds.[14]
- ○ The examiner may report the test as present or absent.[11] In addition, the time (in seconds) the patient is feeling the vibration may be reported.[13,14] Finally, the examiner may compare the vibration sense of the patient compared with themselves.
- • Testing for reflexes (large-nerve fiber) should be done using a reflex hammer.

Steps to perform reflex testing:
- ○ The patient should be instructed to relax.
- ○ The examiner should tap the Achilles tendon while the foot is dorsiflexed.
- ○ If the reflex is absent or difficult to elicit, the examiner may ask the patient to perform reinforcement procedures (eg, asking the patient to clench teeth or hook their fingers together and pull apart)[7]
- ○ If the ankle reflex remains absent, examining the knee reflex is encouraged.

Vascular assessment:

- • The dorsalis pedis and posterior tibial pulses should be examined.
- • Peripheral arterial disease may occur even if the pedal pulses are present. If there is a high index of suspicion, ankle-brachial index testing should be performed.

A Monofilament Test is Insensate to 5.07 but Intact to 6.65. Tuning Fork Vibrations Sense was Lost after Five Seconds. The Ankle Reflex and Pinprick Sensation were Intact Bilaterally. What is the Significance of that Foot Examination?

The importance of performing the foot examination is to identify high-risk patients and to prevent ulceration and amputation. Individuals who are insensate to the 5.07 (10-g) monofilament have a tenfold increased risk of ulceration.[15] The presence of abnormalities in the foot examination may also point to a need to increase the frequency of foot examinations. While the general recommendation for HCP is to examine the healthy feet once yearly, individuals with loss of protective sensation should have a foot examination at least every 3 to 6 months.[7] Individuals with insensate feet may not be able to recognize wounds given the loss of protective sensations; therefore, it is important for patients to examine their feet daily and for HCP to examine the feet at every visit.

What Measures can Health Care Providers do to Prevent Diabetic Symmetric Polyneuropathy and Ulcerations?

Foot care education

Diabetic foot care should be provided to the patient at least at the initial visit and as indicated thereafter and should include the following recommendations[16]:

- Feet should be checked daily. Individuals should look for cuts, redness, swelling, sores, blisters, corns, calluses, or any changes. If the patient cannot see the bottom (plantar aspect) of the foot, a mirror can be used, or a family member can inspect the foot. If none are available, the patient may use their hand as a method to inspect the bottom of the foot.
- Feet should be washed every day in warm, not hot, water. After washing the feet, they should be completely dried particularly between the toes.
- Avoid barefoot walking. Individuals with diabetes should be encouraged to wear socks and shoes outdoors and slippers indoors.
- Shoes should fit well. Patients should be encouraged to always check the inside of the shoes.
- Avoid cutting corns/calluses.
- Toenails should be trimmed straight across.
- Protect the feet from hot and cold. In individuals with insensate feet, it is important to check shower or bath water with the elbow to test the warmth of the water. Patients should be cautious at the beach as sun and sand exposure may result in skin burns.
- Smoking cessation should be encouraged.
- The HCP can guide patients to access publicly available materials: https://www.niddk.nih.gov/health-information/diabetes/overview/preventing-problems/foot-problems and https://www.cdc.gov/diabetes/library/features/healthy-feet.html

Proper footwear

In individuals with increased risk of ulceration, custom-made shoes with inserts are encouraged.[16] If a custom-made shoe is not available or not affordable, cushioned socks are inexpensive and may decrease pressure points.[11]

Glycemic control

Improvement of glycemic control in T1DM has been shown to prevent and delay DSPN. Although the evidence is not as strong in T2DM, improvement in glycemic control may slow the progression of DSPN and is recommended in published guidelines.[17]

Management of Symptomatic Diabetic Symmetric Polyneuropathy

Patients should be offered therapies in a stepwise fashion.[17] Before the initiation of medications, the patient's medication list should be reviewed, and clear goals and expectations should be discussed. In individuals with symptoms impacting the quality of life, pregabalin or duloxetine can be initiated (both have received FDA approval to treat neuropathic pain). If symptoms remain uncontrolled despite adequate titration of one agent, switching to the other agent is recommended.[1,17] If no clinically meaningful effect is observed despite switching to the other agent, combining both pregabalin and duloxetine is recommended.[1] If pregabalin is not affordable, gabapentin may be an acceptable alternative.[17] Pregabalin and gabapentin should be used with caution in older adults and should not be combined. In individuals having neuropathic pain and depression, duloxetine (preferably) or venlafaxine may be favored. In individuals with contraindication(s) to the above medications or unwilling to take oral medications, topical capsaicin, topical lidocaine, or alpha-lipoic acid may be tried.[11] While tapentadol received FDA approval for neuropathic pain, its use should be avoided due to high risk for addiction and limited evidence of benefit.[17]

DIABETIC KIDNEY DISEASE
What is Diabetic Kidney Disease?

The ADA defined diabetic kidney disease (DKD) as chronic kidney disease (CKD) attributed to diabetes, and CKD as the persistent presence of elevated urinary albumin excretion, low estimated glomerular filtration rate (GFR), or other manifestations of kidney damage.[17]

The Kidney Disease: Improving Global Outcomes (KDIGO) guidelines defined CKD as abnormalities of the kidney structure or function present for ≥3 months.[18] In 2007, the KDIGO guidelines recommended using the term "DKD" instead of "diabetic nephropathy" as there is no consensus definition of diabetic nephropathy.[19] In 2020, the KDIGO guidelines used the term "Diabetes and CKD" over "DKD" although DKD was still considered appropriate, to ensure that other causes of CKD are considered and avoid the assumption that all cases of CKD are caused by traditional diabetes pathophysiology.[18]

The Johns Hopkins Diabetes Guide defined DKD as a disease initially characterized by moderately increased urine albumin-to-creatinine ratio (UACR), then severely increased UACR, followed by renal insufficiency, and finally end-stage renal disease (ESRD).[20]

How Common is Diabetic Kidney Disease?

DKD occurs in 20% to 40% of individuals with diabetes.[17] While DKD may be present at the time of diagnosis of T2DM, it usually develops 10 years after the diagnosis of T1DM.[17] DKD remains the leading cause of ESRD in the United States,[17] as more than 50% of individuals on renal replacement therapy have diabetes as the major cause of renal failure.[5]

When should Health Care Providers Initiate Screening for Diabetic Kidney Disease? How Often Should the Screening be Done?

Similar to DSPN, screening for DKD should begin after 5 years from the time of diagnosis of T1DM but at the time of diagnosis of T2DM.[17] In individuals without DKD, annual screening with UACR and creatinine/GFR is recommended. In individuals with DKD, more frequent monitoring is recommended (**Fig. 2**).[17]

How Should the Health Care Providers Interpret the Urine Albumin-to-creatinine Ratio?

- Normal UACR: less than 30 mg/g.
- Moderately increased albuminuria: ≥30 mg/g and ≤300 mg/g.
- Severely increased albuminuria: greater than 300 mg/g.

Given the high biological variability of greater than 20% between measurements, an abnormal UACR requires 2 to 3 abnormal specimens within a 3 to 6 month period. It

CKD is classified based on: • Cause (C) • GFR (G) • Albuminuria (A)				Albuminuria categories Description and range		
				A1	A2	A3
				Normal to mildly increased	Moderately increased	Severely increased
				<30 mg/g <3 mg/mmol	30–299 mg/g 3–29 mg/mmol	≥300 mg/g ≥30 mg/mmol
GFR categories (mL/min/1.73m²) Description and range	G1	Normal to high	≥90	1 If CKD	Treat 1	Refer* 2
	G2	Mildly decreased	60–89	1 If CKD	Treat 1	Refer* 2
	G3a	Mildly to moderately decreased	45–59	Treat 1	Treat 2	Refer 3
	G3b	Moderately to severely decreased	30–44	Treat 2	Treat 3	Refer 3
	G4	Severely decreased	15–29	Refer* 3	Refer* 3	Refer 4+
	G5	Kidney failure	<15	Refer 4+	Refer 4+	Refer 4+

Fig. 2. Frequency of monitoring renal functions in DKD. The numbers in the boxes are a guide to the frequency of visits (number of times/year). (From Chapter 2: Definition, identification, and prediction of CKD progression. Kidney Int Suppl (2011). 2013; 3(1): 63-72; with permission.)

should be noted that the UACR result is also influenced by exercise, infection, fever, congestive heart failure, marked hyperglycemia, marked hypertension, and menstruation.[17]

What is the Likelihood of Diabetic Kidney Disease in Individuals with Moderate/Severe Albuminuria?

Individuals with severely increased albuminuria are likely to have DKD regardless of the GFR.[19] DKD is a possibility in individuals that have CKD3 and moderately increased albuminuria. Individuals with CKD4-5 with moderately increased albuminuria or CKD3-5 with normal albuminuria are unlikely to have DKD, and other etiologies of kidney disease should be explored.[19]

When to Refer to Nephrology?

Referral is recommended for a patient with GFR less than 30 mL/min/1.73 m², rapid worsening of UACR or creatinine/GFR, or an uncertain etiology.[17]

How Should the Health Care Providers Monitor Glycemic Control in Individuals with Diabetic Kidney Disease?

Measurement of blood or interstitial glucose via finger stick blood glucose (FSBG) or continuous glucose monitor (CGM) is likely to be accurate in CKD, dialysis, and kidney transplant.[18] While monitoring of hemoglobin A1c continues to be encouraged in DKD, its reliability is low, particularly in advanced DKD (GFR <30 mL/min/1.73 m²), given the shortened survival of erythrocytes from anemia, transfusions, and use of erythropoiesis-stimulating agents or iron-replacement therapies.[18] The more advanced the kidney disease, the weaker the correlation between FSBG and hemoglobin A1c.[18] Although monitoring glycemic control via hemoglobin A1c remains the currently recommended approach, CGM is expected to limit/eliminate the use of hemoglobin A1c in the future. Taken altogether, if there is a clinical concern that hemoglobin A1c is inaccurate based on discordance with FSBG levels, it is reasonable to either use FSBG or CGM.

What Measures can Reduce the Risk of Developing Diabetic Kidney Disease?

Nutrition
While lower dietary protein intake may slow the progression of CKD, it may be challenging in individuals with diabetes who are encouraged to limit carbohydrates. In addition, protein intake may help individuals on insulin avoid hypoglycemia.[18] Therefore, individuals with DKD not treated with dialysis should maintain a protein intake of 0.8 g/kg/day similar to that of healthy individuals.[18]

Lipid management
Individuals with DKD are at high risk for cardiovascular disease. Statin therapy has been shown to reduce the risk of cardiovascular and kidney disease.[18]

Blood pressure
It is encouraged to target a blood pressure (BP) <130/80 mmHg, particularly in high-risk individuals with albuminuria, if it can be achieved without complications. In those who cannot achieve a BP <130/80 mmHg, a less strict goal of less than 140/90 mmHg can be recommended.[17]

Glycemic control
Adequate glycemic control may be key to preventing microvascular complications, including DKD; however, targets should be individualized. While a lower hemoglobin A1c target of less than 7.0% may be key in preventing complications, a higher hemoglobin A1c target (<8.0%) might be preferred in individuals with established comorbidities or if they are at increased risk of hypoglycemia.[17,18]

Smoking
Counseling for smoking cessation should be provided.

A 55-year-old Individual with T2DM Treated with Metformin. His Last Creatinine was 1.7 mg/dL, GFR 51 mL/min/1.73 m², and UACR 389 mg/g. Should Metformin be Discontinued?

The ADA standards of management recommend the initiation and titration of metformin if GFR is $\geq$45 mL/min/1.73 m², to continue use if GFR falls to less than 45 mL/min/1.73 m² after reassessing benefits and risk, and to discontinue metformin if GFR is <30 mL/min/1.73 m². While the KDIGO guidelines similarly recommend metformin without restrictions when GFR is $\geq$45 mL/min/1.73 m², it recommends halving the dose (if already on metformin) or initiating metformin at half the dose and titrating upwards to half of the maximum dose (if not previously on metformin) if the GFR is between 30 to 45 mL/min/1.73 m².[18] In individuals with renal transplant, metformin can be used as long as the GFR is $\geq$30 mL/min/1.73 m².[18]

How can Health Care Providers Delay Progression of Diabetic Kidney Disease?

Renin–angiotensin system blockade
The use of a renin–angiotensin system (RAS) blocking agent is recommended as the initial drug of choice in DKD. In individuals with diabetes, hypertension, and albuminuria, RAS blockade, resulting from agents such as angiotensin-converting enzyme inhibitors (ACEi) or angiotensin II receptor blockers (ARBs), should be initiated and titrated to the highest approved dose that is tolerated.[18] In individuals with diabetes

and albuminuria but without hypertension, treatment with an ACEi or ARB may be considered.[18] It is recommended to follow-up with a repeat serum potassium and serum creatinine measurements in 2 to 4 weeks after the initiation of ACEi or ARB and to continue use unless the creatinine rise is greater than 30%. If hyperkalemia is noted, the dose of ACEi or ARB may need to be reduced.[18] The combination of ACEi and ARB should be avoided as side effects may be more pronounced.

Sodium–glucose co-transporter-2 inhibitors

In the renal outcome trials, dapagliflozin (DAPA-CKD)[21] and canagliflozin (CREDENCE)[22] showed a significantly lower risk of renal disease worsening. In individuals with DKD, sodium–glucose co-transporter-2 inhibitors (SGLT-2i) should be considered to reduce cardiovascular risk and to delay progression to ESRD provided that GFR is $\geq$25 to 30 mL/min/1.73 m^2 (although continuation with lower GFR is recommended and initiation at lower GFR may be evaluated in the future).[17] While SGLT-2i should be encouraged in DKD, it remains debatable in T1DM given the increased risk for diabetic ketoacidosis. Patients should be educated to withhold SGLT-2is if they cannot maintain adequate hydration (such as before surgery or if sick). In individuals on other diuretics who are at risk for hypovolemia, reducing the dose of diuretic may be reasonable, and close follow-up is encouraged.

What Anti-diabetic Medications Should be Added if Glycemic Control is not Achieved by Metformin and Sodium–glucose Co-transporter-2 Inhibitors?

Glucagon-like peptide-1 receptor agonists (GLP-1RA) may be a preferred agent given the known cardiovascular benefit and possible kidney benefit.[18] If GLP-1RA cannot be used, pioglitazone may be considered, as it delays cardio-renal disease progression. However, pioglitazone should be used with caution as it can cause fluid overload and unmask heart failure.[23,24]

Novel Therapy in Diabetic Kidney Disease

Mineralocorticoid receptor antagonists: In FIDELIO-DKD,[25] patients treated with finerenone had a significant reduction in CKD progression and cardiovascular events. Hyperkalemia remains a concern, particularly when added to RAS blockade. Nevertheless, this may be an option for add-on therapy in the future. This may be specifically beneficial in individuals with DKD and hypertension.[17,18]

DIABETIC RETINOPATHY
What is Diabetic Retinopathy?

The most common diabetes-related eye disease is diabetic retinopathy (DR). DR is characterized by a gradually progressive alteration in the retinal microvasculature resulting in areas of retinal nonperfusion with a resultant increase in vascular endothelial growth factor-A (VEGF). Elevated levels of VEGF can result in abnormal development of new blood vessels (neovascularization). Those new vessels can be friable and bleed into the vitreous cavity, causing vitreous hemorrhage. Vision-threatening DR develops in about 10% of people with diabetes and remains the leading cause of new cases of legal blindness.[26]

When Should Screening Begin and How Frequently Should Testing be Done?

Screening should be performed by an ophthalmologist or optometrist within 5 years from diagnosis of T1DM but at the time of diagnosis of T2DM.[17,27] The eye examination is needed annually for the first 2 years, then every 2 years if no retinopathy is noted and adequate glycemic control has been achieved.[17] Individuals with diagnosed DR may be followed more frequently.[27] If there is limited access to ophthalmologists or optometrists (eg, in rural communities), digital retinal photography with remote reading may be an option to improve access to ophthalmologic evaluation.[27–29]

Are Pregnant Women Screened Similarly?

Pregnancy can exacerbate DR. Ideally, women planning to become pregnant should have a comprehensive eye examination within 1 year before conception and then again in each trimester.[5,17]

How Should the Health Care Providers Classify Diabetic Retinopathy?

- No apparent DR[30]
- Nonproliferative DR (NPDR): Can be further classified into mild (microaneurysms only), moderate (microaneurysms, blot hemorrhages, hard exudates, cotton wool spots but less than severe), and severe (intraretinal hemorrhages, venous beading) (**Fig. 3**).[30]
- Proliferative DR (PDR): Presence of neovascularization or vitreous/preretinal hemorrhage (**Fig. 4**).[30]

Diabetic macular edema (DME) can develop at any stage of DR. This disease is classified into no DME (no retinal thickening in the macula), noncenter involving DME (retinal thickening in the macula that does not involve the central zone), and center-involving DME (retinal thickening in the macular that involves the central zone that is 1 mm in diameter).

What is the Role of the Health Care Providers in Preventing/Treating Diabetic Retinopathy?

Ensure regular eye examination
Many individuals with DME are not aware that diabetes has affected their eyes, and many with PDR have not been examined by an ophthalmologist within the last 2 years.[5]

Hyperglycemia
The longer the duration of hyperglycemia and the worse the glycemic control, the greater the risk for developing DR.[27] Lowering hemoglobin A1c has been shown to prevent and delay the progression of DR. A target hemoglobin A1c <7.0% is considered ideal; however, any reduction in hemoglobin A1c can be beneficial.[27] It should be noted that the rapid correction of long-standing hyperglycemia may be associated with transient worsening of retinopathy. While any antidiabetic medication can be used, pioglitazone and semaglutide should be used with caution as DME was reported in individuals on pioglitazone and worsening retinopathy may be associated with semaglutide, although more research is needed.

Blood pressure control
Achieving a systolic blood pressure of less than 130 mmHg has been shown to slow the progression of DR. While controlling the blood pressure reduces retinopathy, the use of RAS inhibitors specifically has been shown to reduce the incidence and risk of progression of DR.[31]

Lipid control
Treatment with the peroxisome proliferative-activated receptor gamma (PPAR-α) agonist, fenofibrate, reduced the risk of progression by up to 40% among patients with NPDR.[31]

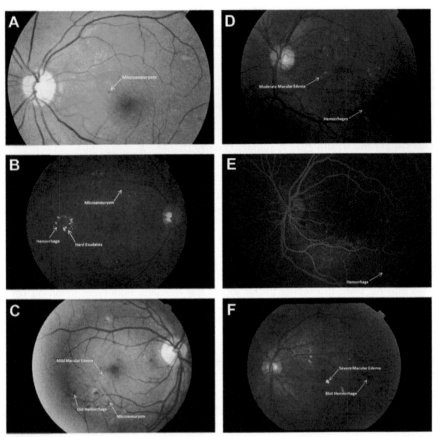

Fig. 3. Features of mild and moderate to severe stages of NPDR. (*A*) Fundus photograph showing mild NPDR with microaneurysms. (*B*) Fundus photograph showing moderate NPDR with hemorrhages, hard exudates, and microaneurysms. (*C*) Fundus photograph showing moderate NPDR with mild DME. (*D*) Fundus photograph showing moderate macular edema. (*E*) Fluorescein angiogram showing moderate NPDR with non–center-involving DME. (*F*) Fundus photograph showing severe NPDR with center-involving DME. (*From* Wong TY, Sun J, Kawasaki R, Ruamviboonsuk P, Gupta N, Lansingh VC, Maia M, Mathenge W, Moreker S, Muqit MMK, Resnikoff S, Verdaguer J, Zhao P, Ferris F, Aiello LP, Taylor HR. Guidelines on Diabetic Eye Care: The International Council of Ophthalmology Recommendations for Screening, Follow-up, Referral, and Treatment Based on Resource Settings. Ophthalmology. 2018 Oct; 125(10): 1608-1622; with permission.)

Lifestyle modifications

Regular exercise is encouraged in individuals with or without retinopathy, as it may prevent and/or delay the progression of retinopathy. In individuals with PDR, activities resulting in a Valsalva maneuver should be avoided as they may result in vitreous hemorrhage. Smoking cessation should be encouraged in individuals who smoke.

What are the Treatment Options for Diabetic Retinopathy?

If the measures above fail to prevent or control DR, laser photocoagulation and anti-VEGF therapy may be used for treatment. Pan-retinal laser photocoagulation is used to treat high-risk PDR and occasionally for severe NPDR.[30] While pan-retinal laser photocoagulation is still commonly used to manage PDR, the use of anti-VEGF

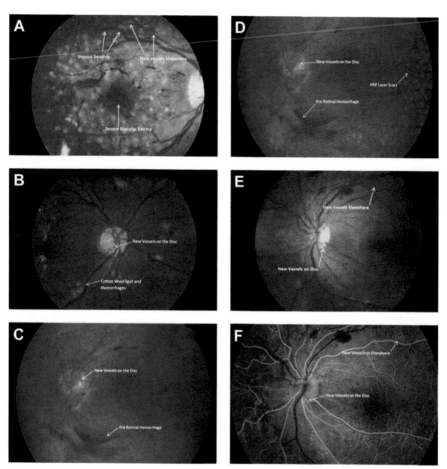

Fig. 4. Features of severe stages of PDR and DME. (*A*) Fundus photograph showing PDR with venous beading, new vessels elsewhere, and severe DME. (*B*) Fundus photograph showing high-risk PDR with new vessels at the disc. (*C*) Fundus photograph showing high-risk PDR with preretinal hemorrhage and new vessels on the disc. (*D*) Fundus photograph showing high-risk PDR with new panretinal photocoagulation (PRP) scars. (*E*) Fundus photograph showing PDR. New vessels seem on the disc and elsewhere. (*F*) Fluorescein angiogram showing PDR. New vessels seem on the disc and elsewhere. (*From* Wong TY, Sun J, Kawasaki R, Ruamviboonsuk P, Gupta N, Lansingh VC, Maia M, Mathenge W, Moreker S, Muqit MMK, Resnikoff S, Verdaguer J, Zhao P, Ferris F, Aiello LP, Taylor HR. Guidelines on Diabetic Eye Care: The International Council of Ophthalmology Recommendations for Screening, Follow-up, Referral, and Treatment Based on Resource Settings. Ophthalmology. 2018 Oct; 125(10): 1608-1622; with permission.)

therapy was associated with a rapid regression of retinal neovascularization.[27,30] Anti-VEGF agents are the current standard of care for central-involved DME.[27]

SUMMARY

In summary, microvascular complications including DSPN, DKD, and DR are common in patients with long-standing type 1 diabetes and new or existing type 2 diabetes and require active screening. Complications can be prevented or delayed by careful attention to risk factors, careful education and monitoring by the patient, and prompt evaluation and treatment by consultants when indicated. This evaluation, monitoring, prevention, and treatment can help improve patients' quality of life and can be associated with reductions or delays in treatments such as dialysis with reduced cost.

CLINICS CARE POINTS

- Screening for diabetes-related microvascular complications should start immediately at the time of diagnosis of T2DM and within 5 years after the diagnosis of T1DM.

DSPN:

- Screening for DSPN is essential as around 50% of individuals with DSPN are asymptomatic and will not volunteer symptoms.
- Before diagnosing DSPN, HCP may need to rule out other causes of neuropathy.
- In clinical practice, nerve conduction studies and skin biopsy are rarely indicated.
- In individuals with DSPN, an annual foot examination may not be adequate and exam/inspection at every visit is suggested.
- Patients should be encouraged to check their feet daily.
- Foot care education should be provided to the patient at least at the initial visit and as indicated.
- In individuals who are at high risk for ulceration and amputations, HCP should prescribe diabetic shoes and consider a podiatry referral.

DKD:

- In individuals without DKD, annual serum creatinine and UACR are required.
- An abnormal UACR requires 2 to 3 abnormal specimens within a 3- to 6-month period to confirm the diagnosis of albuminuria.
- If the GFR is < 30 mL/min/1.73 m^2, there is a rapid worsening of renal functions, or the etiology is unclear, the patient should be referred to nephrology.
- The reliability of hemoglobin A1c is low in advanced DKD.
- In individuals with DKD, RAS blockade agent and/or SGLT-2i are recommended. Finerenone can reduce CKD progression and cardiovascular events.

DR:

- An eye examination by an expert is needed at least annually for the first 2 years.
- Individuals with diagnosed DR may require a more frequent monitoring schedule.
- Digital retinal photography with remote reading may be an option in locations with limited access to ophthalmologic evaluation.
- In patients seeking pregnancy, a comprehensive eye examination within 1 year before conception and then during pregnancy is indicated as pregnancy may exacerbate DR.
- The use of RAS inhibitor has shown to reduce the incidence and risk of progression of DR.

DISCLOSURE

BMM has served on Advisory Board Panels for AstraZeneca and Bayer with the consulting fees paid directly to East Carolina University. BMM also received a research grant (to East Carolina University) from Eli Lilly and Company.
DMC and JRP report no conflict of interest.

REFERENCES

1. Pop-Busui R, Boulton AJ, Feldman EL, et al. Diabetic neuropathy: a position statement by the American Diabetes Association. Diabetes Care 2017;40(1): 136–54.
2. Feldman EL, Callaghan BC, Pop-Busui R, et al. Diabetic neuropathy. Nat Rev Dis Primers 2019;5(1):41.
3. England JD, Gronseth GS, Franklin G, et al. Distal symmetric polyneuropathy: a definition for clinical research: report of the American Academy of Neurology, the American Association of Electrodiagnostic Medicine, and the American Academy of Physical Medicine and Rehabilitation. Neurology 2005;64(2):199–207.
4. England JD, Gronseth GS, Franklin G, et al. Practice parameter: evaluation of distal symmetric polyneuropathy: role of autonomic testing, nerve biopsy, and skin biopsy (an evidence-based review). Report of the American Academy of Neurology, American Association of Neuromuscular and Electrodiagnostic Medicine, and American Academy of Physical Medicine and Rehabilitation. Neurology 2009;72(2):177–84.
5. Brownlee M, Aiello LP, Cooper ME, et al. Complications of diabetes mellitus. In: Williams Textbook of Endocrinology. 13th edition; 2016. p. 1484.
6. Vinik AI, Nevoret ML, Casellini C, et al. Diabetic neuropathy. Endocrinol Metab Clin North Am 2013;42(4):747–87.
7. Boulton AJ, Armstrong DG, Albert SF, et al. Comprehensive foot examination and risk assessment: a report of the task force of the foot care interest group of the American Diabetes Association, with endorsement by the American Association of Clinical Endocrinologists. Diabetes Care 2008;31(8):1679–85.
8. Feng Y, Schlösser FJ, Sumpio BE. The Semmes Weinstein monofilament examination as a screening tool for diabetic peripheral neuropathy. J Vasc Surg 2009;50(3):675–82, 682.e1.
9. Jeng C, Michelson J, Mizel M. Sensory thresholds of normal human feet. Foot Ankle Int 2000;21(6):501–4.
10. Olaiya MT, Hanson RL, Kavena KG, et al. Use of graded Semmes Weinstein monofilament testing for ascertaining peripheral neuropathy in people with and without diabetes. Diabetes Res Clin Pract 2019;151:1–10.
11. Tanenberg R, Donofrio PD. Neuropathic problems of the lower limbs in diabetic patietns. In: The diabetic foot. 7th edition; 2008. p. 33–40.
12. Miller JD, Carter E, Shih J, et al. How to do a 3-minute diabetic foot exam. J Fam Pract 2014;63(11):646–56.
13. Takahara M, Fujiwara Y, Sakamoto F, et al. Assessment of vibratory sensation with a tuning fork at different sites in Japanese patients with diabetes mellitus. J Diabetes Invest 2014;5(1):90–3.
14. Prabhakar AT, Suresh T, Kurian DS, et al. Timed vibration sense and joint position sense testing in the diagnosis of distal sensory polyneuropathy. J Neurosci Rural Pract 2019;10(2):273–7.
15. Thomson MP, Potter J, Finch PM, et al. Threshold for detection of diabetic peripheral sensory neuropathy using a range of research grade monofilaments in persons with Type 2 diabetes mellitus. J Foot Ankle Res 2008;1(1):9.
16. van Netten JJ, Lazzarini PA, Armstrong DG, et al. Diabetic foot Australia guideline on footwear for people with diabetes. J Foot Ankle Res 2018;11:2.
17. American Diabetes Association. 11. Microvascular complications and foot care: standards of medical care in diabetes-2021. Diabetes Care 2021;44(Suppl 1): S151–67.

18. KDIGO 2020 clinical practice guideline for diabetes management in chronic kidney disease. Kidney Int 2020;98(4s):S1–115.
19. KDOQI clinical practice guidelines and clinical practice recommendations for diabetes and chronic kidney disease. Am J Kidney Dis 2007;49(Suppl 2): S12–154.
20. Knicely DH, Myers D. Diabetic kidney disease. Johns Hopkins Diabetes Guide; 2019. Johns Hopkins Guide. Available at: www.hopkinsguides.com/hopkins/view/Johns_Hopkins_Diabetes_Guide/547097/all/Diabetic_Kidney_Disease. July 4, 2021.
21. Heerspink HJL, Stefánsson BV, Correa-Rotter R, et al. Dapagliflozin in patients with chronic kidney disease. N Engl J Med 2020;383(15):1436–46.
22. Perkovic V, Jardine MJ, Neal B, et al. Canagliflozin and renal outcomes in type 2 diabetes and nephropathy. N Engl J Med 2019;380(24):2295–306.
23. DeFronzo RA, Inzucchi S, Abdul-Ghani M, et al. Pioglitazone: the forgotten, cost-effective cardioprotective drug for type 2 diabetes. Diabetes Vasc Dis Res 2019; 16(2):133–43.
24. Schneider CA, Ferrannini E, Defronzo R, et al. Effect of pioglitazone on cardiovascular outcome in diabetes and chronic kidney disease. J Am Soc Nephrol 2008; 19(1):182–7.
25. Bakris GL, Agarwal R, Anker SD, et al. Effect of finerenone on chronic kidney disease outcomes in type 2 diabetes. N Engl J Med 2020;383(23):2219–29.
26. Yau JW, Rogers SL, Kawasaki R, et al. Global prevalence and major risk factors of diabetic retinopathy. Diabetes Care 2012;35(3):556–64.
27. Solomon SD, Chew E, Duh EJ, et al. Diabetic retinopathy: a position statement by the American Diabetes Association. Diabetes Care 2017;40(3):412–8.
28. Cummings DM, Morrissey S, Barondes MJ, et al. Screening for diabetic retinopathy in rural areas: the potential of telemedicine. J Rural Health 2001;17(1):25–31.
29. Newman R, Cummings DM, Doherty L, et al. Digital retinal imaging in a residency-based patient-centered medical home. Fam Med 2012;44(3):159–63.
30. Wong TY, Sun J, Kawasaki R, et al. Guidelines on diabetic eye care: the international council of ophthalmology recommendations for screening, follow-up, referral, and treatment based on resource settings. Ophthalmology 2018; 125(10):1608–22.
31. Antonetti DA, Klein R, Gardner TW. Diabetic retinopathy. N Engl J Med 2012; 366(13):1227–39.

Macrovascular Complications

Michael McRae, DO[a], Cecilia C. Low Wang, MD[b],*

KEYWORDS

- Diabetes • Atherosclerotic cardiovascular disease • Heart failure
- Cardiovascular outcome trial • Risk factor modification

KEY POINTS

- Atherosclerotic cardiovascular disease (ASCVD) is a leading cause of morbidity and mortality in individuals with diabetes mellitus.
- ASCVD includes not just coronary artery disease but also heart failure, peripheral artery disease, cerebrovascular disease, and coronary heart disease.
- Lifestyle modifications including a healthy eating pattern, physical activity, and moderate weight loss if overweight or obese are cornerstones of cardiovascular risk reduction.
- Strong clinical trial evidence supports the use of statin and PCSK9i, glucagon-like peptide 1 receptor agonists (GLP1RA), and sodium/glucose cotransporter-2 inhibitors (SGLT2i) therapy for patients with diabetes and established or at high risk for ASCVD; GLP1RA reduce risk of major adverse cardiovascular (CV) events, and most SGLT2i reduce risk of heart failure hospitalizations and CV death.
- Low-dose aspirin, icosapent ethyl, and rivaroxaban are recommended for patients with established ASCVD and selected patients for primary prevention.

INTRODUCTION

Cardiovascular disease is the leading cause of death and decreased quality of life in individuals with diabetes in the United States.[1] Persons with type 2 diabetes die 14.6 years earlier than those without diabetes.[2] Approximately 66% of deaths in type 2 diabetes are related to cardiovascular disease (CVD), with 40% specifically resulting from ischemic causes.[3] Macrovascular complications are responsible for the largest proportion of health care costs related to diabetes, making up approximately 85% of diabetes-specific costs or $37.3 billion annually.[1,4] For these reasons, prevention and reduction in risk of macrovascular complications are of paramount importance.

[a] St. Luke's Family Medicine, 9850 W. St. Luke's Drive Suite 290, Nampa, ID 83687, USA;
[b] Department of Medicine, Division of Endocrinology, Metabolism and Diabetes, Anschutz Medical Campus School of Medicine, 12801 East 17th Avenue MS8106, RC-1 South Room 7103, Aurora, CO 80045, USA
* Corresponding author.
E-mail address: Cecilia.Lowwang@cuanschutz.edu

Prim Care Clin Office Pract 49 (2022) 255–273
https://doi.org/10.1016/j.pop.2021.11.012
0095-4543/22/© 2021 Elsevier Inc. All rights reserved.

primarycare.theclinics.com

Macrovascular disease encompasses atherosclerotic cardiovascular disease (ASCVD) and includes any coronary artery disease, coronary heart disease, cerebrovascular disease, peripheral artery disease, and congestive heart failure (HF) presumed to be of atherosclerotic cause. Raising awareness and implementation of lifestyle changes are crucial to improving cardiovascular outcomes. Strong evidence supports cholesterol lowering with statins and control of blood pressure as methods of improving these outcomes. Selected patients should receive antiplatelet therapy with aspirin, whereas others may be candidates for antithrombotic therapy. Our toolbox for CVD prevention and risk reduction now includes most of the medications in 2 newer classes of antihyperglycemic agents—glucagon-like peptide-1 receptor agonists (GLP1RA) and sodium glucose cotransporter-2 inhibitors (SGLT2i)—and have been demonstrated in large clinical cardiovascular outcome trials (CVOT) to reduce the risk of macrovascular complications in diabetes. This new evidence for ASCVD risk reduction is associated with a significant decline in CVD risk among patients with diabetes in the past couple of decades, but, unfortunately, the relative and overall risks remain high.[5]

All clinicians caring for individuals with diabetes can take vital steps toward helping reduce risk for CVD by identifying those individuals who would benefit from specific medical therapies and raising awareness in individuals at particularly high CVD risk. These individuals include, but are not limited to, those with hyperlipidemia, hypertension, uncontrolled glycemia, albuminuria, family history of early heart disease, certain ethnic groups, especially those at lower body mass index (BMI) such as South Asians and East Asians, and women with a history of gestational diabetes, preeclampsia, and/or metabolic syndrome. Unfortunately, we still have a lot of work to do, with only 14.3% of Americans with type 2 diabetes having achieved goal levels for hemoglobin A1c, blood pressure, and cholesterol.[6] Equipped with accurate and up-to-date information regarding the evidence, and a clear understanding of potential benefits and risks of these therapies, clinicians can make a huge impact to help reduce the incidence of macrovascular complications in their patients with diabetes.

Despite the increased risk of CVD in diabetes, there is no benefit for screening asymptomatic patients with diabetes using electrocardiograms or stress testing.[7,8] Symptomatic individuals, however, should be screened appropriately. All patients with diabetes should receive recommendations for evidence-based lifestyle changes and optimal medical therapy to minimize risk of ASCVD.

This section discusses key evidence and recommendations for macrovascular disease risk reduction in diabetes patients.

LIFESTYLE INTERVENTIONS AND WEIGHT LOSS

Lifestyle interventions should be at the forefront of discussions with patients regarding how best to prevent macrovascular complications in diabetes. Arguably, weight loss through a healthy lifestyle has the greatest impact on all metabolic diseases including diabetes. The weight loss goal should be patient centered. As little as 5% weight loss has been demonstrated to result in metabolic improvement and CV risk reduction,[9,10] and greater degree of weight loss allows for deescalation of antihyperglycemic and other therapies and may lead to diabetes remission. For example, the Diabetes Remission Clinical Trial (DiRECT) recruited patients with type 2 diabetes for less than 6 years who were not on insulin therapy to determine whether a structured, intensive weight loss program in a primary care setting would be a viable treatment to achieve durable normoglycemia.[11] The DiRECT intervention resulted in 86% of patients achieving weight loss of more than 15 kg and experiencing diabetes remission at 12 months.[11]

Physical activity is strongly associated with reduction in CVD risk in patients with diabetes. A meta-analysis of 17 studies demonstrated that individuals with the highest physical activity levels had a 29% lower relative risk of CVD and 39% lower relative risk for all-cause mortality than those with the lowest physical activity level.[12] There was a dose-response relationship between physical activity and CVD risk, and any amount of habitual physical activity was better than inactivity. Physical activity alone is generally not sufficient to result in weight loss, but regular physical activity is an essential component of a healthy lifestyle to improve metabolic health.

Bariatric surgery results in significant weight loss and reduction in risk of macrovascular and microvascular complications of diabetes.[13,14] Indications for weight loss surgery include BMI greater than 40 kg/m^2 (37.5 kg/m^2 for Asian Americans) or greater than 35 kg/m^2 with comorbidities (>32.5 kg/m^2 for Asian Americans) and inability to achieve and/or maintain weight loss through lifestyle interventions and/or medications.[10] Diabetes remission after bariatric surgery is most likely in patients earlier in the disease process, with shorter duration of diabetes.[15]

There are several medications approved by the Food and Drug Administration (FDA) for weight loss. Of these, many of the GLP1RA have strong evidence to support CV risk reduction, but lorcaserin was not demonstrated to result in CV risk reduction after a median of 3.3 years of follow-up, and CV outcomes have not been studied for other weight-loss medications.[16]

GLYCEMIC CONTROL

Glucose lowering has a modest effect to reduce CV risk, ranging from 11% to 16% for every 1% decrease in A1c in individuals with type 2 diabetes in the United Kingdom Prospective Diabetes Study (UKPDS)[17,18] and 42% reduction in risk of any CVD over 17 years as observed in the Diabetes Control and Complications Trial/Epidemiology of Diabetes Interventions and Complications (DCCT/EDIC) trial of patients with type 1 diabetes.[19] The initial analysis of the UKPDS did not demonstrate a statistically significant degree of cardiovascular risk reduction with intensive glycemic control,[20] but risk reductions for myocardial infarction and all-cause mortality emerged in the intensive control group after 10 years of posttrial follow-up.[18] Individuals with type 1 or type 2 diabetes who maintain excellent glycemic control during the first 6 to 7 years of diagnosis continue to experience lower vascular risk from this period of good glycemic control even decades later, a phenomenon referred to as "metabolic memory" or the "legacy effect."[18,19,21]

CVOT conducted since the 2008 guidance by the FDA for evaluation of CV risk of new antidiabetes agents have consistently demonstrated CV safety of the new agents with a few exceptions and resulted in significant changes in diabetes clinical practice. There was surprising and strong evidence for CV risk reduction demonstrated for several agents in the GLP1RA and SGLT2i drug classes. The most recent Standards of Medical Care for Diabetes by the American Diabetes Association (ADA) recommends that metformin remain the initial drug of choice along with lifestyle changes due to its low cost and effectiveness for glycemic control as well as its use as baseline therapy in all of the CVOT.[22] However, individuals with established or at high risk for ASCVD, HF particularly with reduced left ventricular ejection fraction (HFrEF), and/or chronic kidney disease (CKD) should receive an antidiabetes agent demonstrated to reduce risk or progression of CV, HF, and/or CKD regardless of the patient's A1c target, A1c value, or metformin use.[23]

CARDIOVASCULAR RISK REDUCTION WITH ANTIHYPERGLYCEMIC AGENTS

For patients with known ASCVD, a GLP1RA or SGLT2i with proven CV protection is strongly recommended[23] (**Table 1**). GLP1RA medications with evidence for CV risk reduction include liraglutide (SQ daily: Victoza), semaglutide (SQ weekly: Ozempic), and dulaglutide (SQ weekly: Trulicity). Oral semaglutide (PO daily: Rybelsus) is the only oral GLP1RA currently available and unfortunately did not reduce CV risk when studied in the PIONEER-6 trial.[24] The number needed to treat (NNT) to prevent major adverse cardiovascular events (MACE; a composite of nonfatal myocardial infarction, nonfatal stroke, and cardiovascular death) in the major GLP1RA cardiovascular outcome trials for liraglutide (LEADER), semaglutide (SUSTAIN-6), and dulaglutide (REWIND) were 53 (median follow-up of 3.8 years), 43 (follow-up of 2.1 years), and 71 (median follow-up 5.4 years), respectively.[23,25,26] In order to accurately apply clinical trial results when caring for the individual patient, it is essential to keep in mind the baseline characteristics of the trial population (often depicted in "**Table 1**" of the publication). In the CV trials examining liraglutide and semaglutide, more than 80% of patients had established ASCVD at baseline, whereas only 32% of patients in the CV trial examining dulaglutide had established ASCVD, making the results of this last trial more generalizable as a primary prevention strategy. Based on these data, the ADA recommends that GLP1RA be the first-line injected therapy (before insulin) unless patients have signs of insulin deficiency (eg, catabolism, blood glucose >300 or symptoms of hyperglycemia such as significant polydipsia/polyuria), HbA1c greater than 10% or in whom the diagnosis of type 1 diabetes may be a possibility; in these situations, insulin therapy should be strongly considered.[22] GLP1RA agents other than those discussed earlier have not been shown to decrease risk of CVD.[23] A summary of key characteristics of CVOT for each of these agents is detailed in **Table 1**.

The SGLT2i with demonstrated CV risk reduction include empagliflozin, canagliflozin, and dapagliflozin, but the specific CV effects vary depending on the specific agent.[23] The EMPA-REG OUTCOME trial of empagliflozin demonstrated a significant reduction in the primary MACE outcome, but this was driven by a reduction in CV death (38% relative risk reduction). The relative risk of heart failure hospitalization and all-cause mortality was also significantly reduced (35% and 32%, respectively), so empagliflozin has an indication for lowering risk of CV death and hospitalization for heart failure in individuals with type 2 diabetes and established CVD or who are at high CV risk.[27] The CANagliflozin cardioVascular Assessment Study (CANVAS)-1 and -2 trials of canagliflozin, which are usually combined into the "CANVAS program" when results are discussed, demonstrated a 14% reduction in risk of MACE but an increased risk of amputations, mostly below the ankle; however, this amputation signal has not been seen in subsequent trials or in other SGLT2i trials. EMPA-REG OUTCOME included mostly (>99%) patients with established ASCVD, whereas 66% of patients in the CANVAS program had known CVD, and only approximately 40% of patients in the dapagliflozin CVOT (DECLARE-TIMI 58) had established ASCVD.[27–30] A meta-analysis of SGLT2i CVOTs revealed a 14% reduction in relative risk of all-cause mortality with canagliflozin, empagliflozin, and dapagliflozin.[31] However, the newest agent in this class, ertugliflozin, was not demonstrated to reduce risk of CVD in the major CVOT (VERTIS-CV) but resulted in a 30% reduction in the secondary endpoint of hospitalization for heart failure.[31,32] Sotagliflozin is an SGLT2i that has been approved for use in Europe for type 2 diabetes and type 1 diabetes, but not the United States and may have a role in treating patients with CKD or after acute heart failure exacerbation.[23]

Table 1
Antihyperglycemic therapies demonstrated to reduce cardiovascular disease risk

	Dosing	Established ASCVD (%) in CVOT	Duration of CVOT	MACE[a]	CV Death	HHF
GLP1RA						
Liraglutide (Victoza)	SQ QD	~81	3.8 y	13% reduction	22% reduction	NS
Semaglutide (Ozempic)	SQ Qwk	83	2.1 y	26% reduction	NS	NS
Dulaglutide (Trulicity)	SQ Qwk	31	5.4 y	12% reduction	NS	NS
SGLT2i						
Empagliflozin (Jardiance)	PO QD	99	2.6 y	14% reduction	38% reduction	35% reduction
Canagliflozin (Invokana)	PO QD	72	2.4 y[b]	14% reduction	NS	33% reduction
Dapagliflozin (Farxiga)	PO QD	40	4.2 y	NS	[a]Coprimary: CV death or HHF: 17% reduction, driven by HHF	
Ertugliflozin (Steglatro)	PO QD	100	3.0 y[c]	NS	NS	30% reduction

Abbreviations: HHF, hospitalization for heart failure; NS, nonsignificant.

[a] Denotes primary endpoint.
[b] Median follow-up 126 weeks; mean follow-up 188.2 weeks: length of follow-up was similar in the canagliflozin and placebo groups but longer in CANVAS (296 weeks) than in CANVAS-R (108 weeks).
[c] Median duration of follow-up was 3 years (4.6 years in cohort 1 and 2.7 years in cohort 2); mean duration of follow-up was 3.5 years (4.3 years in cohort 1 and 2.7 years in cohort 2).

Although the large CVOT for SGLT2i and GLP1RA included patients with established ASCVD as well as patients without established ASCVD (but were considered high risk), subgroup analyses suggest that the benefit of ASCVD risk reduction is mainly in the subgroup with established ASCVD or secondary prevention. Meta-analyses of SGLT2i and GLP1RA CVOTs support this.[33,34] The exception is dulaglutide (Trulicity), which was studied in the REWIND trial[35] in which only about 32% of patients had established ASCVD and demonstrated a 12% reduction in MACE over a mean follow-up period of 5.4 years. The risk reduction was driven by a decrease in nonfatal strokes but not myocardial infarction or CV death.[23,35] For dapagliflozin, around 60% of patients did not have established ASCVD, and although there was a significant reduction in the coprimary endpoint of hospitalization for heart failure or CV death (driven by 27% reduction in the risk of hospitalization for heart failure), there was no reduction in MACE or CV death.[30] Please refer to **Table 1** for important details from these trials.

The ADA recommends that patients with evidence of ASCVD (left ventricular hypertrophy or those older than 55 years with carotid, coronary, and/or peripheral artery disease) be treated with either an SGLT2i or GLP1RA regardless of HbA1c. On the other hand, if a patient does not have congestive heart failure, CKD, or ASCVD, then there is no preference among dipeptidyl peptidase-4 inhibitors (DPP4i), GLP1RA, pioglitazone, or SGLT2i after metformin.[22] Therefore, it is important to be aware that starting these newer agents solely for primary CV protection in patients without established ASCVD or without risk factors as defined in the CVOTs is not warranted at this time. However, other benefits of GLP1RA and SGLT2i must also be considered, including weight loss, kidney protection, glycemic control, blood pressure reduction, and reduction in hospitalization for heart failure (the latter specifically in SGLT2i).

ANTIHYPERGLYCEMIC AGENTS IN HEART FAILURE

The SGLT2i class of antihyperglycemic agents consistently reduces risk of hospitalization for heart failure in patients with HFrEF (<45%) to a significant degree, with an NNT of 27[36]; this seems to be independent of the diuretic effects of these agents.[37] Diabetes patients with HF should not be started on the DPP4i saxagliptin, which was demonstrated to increase risk of hospitalization for heart failure, whereas thiazolidinediones (pioglitazone and rosiglitazone) should not be used in patients with symptomatic heart failure.[38] In addition, all-cause mortality was significantly reduced in patients with HFrEF in the DAPA-HF trial (NNT 43), which included patients with or without diabetes followed for a median of 18.2 months.[36] Dapagliflozin has also been examined in patients with CKD with or without diabetes and shown to result in renal benefits.[39] Recent data demonstrate a reduction in CV death or hospitalization for heart failure with empagliflozin in patients with heart failure with preserved ejection fraction (EMPEROR-Preserved, NCT03057951), and a clinical trial is ongoing with dapagliflozin (NCT03619213). In summary, patients with type 2 diabetes and established or at high risk of ASCVD should be placed on a proven SGLT2i regardless of metformin use or HbA1c.

CHRINIC KIDNEY DISEASE MANAGEMENT IN CARDIOVASCULAR PROTECTION

CKD is stratified by estimated glomerular filtration rate, and patients with diabetes and CKD are further risk stratified according to the presence or absence of albuminuria. Albuminuria in the setting of CKD is a significant, independent risk factor for CVD and should be treated aggressively. When albuminuria is present, an SGLT2i should be used because there is strong evidence for reduction in the rate of renal decline and development of end-stage renal disease (ESRD).[39,40] Treatment of elevated blood pressure with angiotensin-converting enzyme inhibitor (ACEi) or angiotensin receptor blocker (ARB) therapy decreases the rate of decline in renal function and albuminuria in types 1 or 2 diabetes when patients have severely increased albuminuria,[41–43] with trials showing clear benefit (severely increased albuminuria was previously known as macroalbuminuria or microalbumin/creatinine ratio of >300 mcg/mg).[44,45] The evidence is not as strong for halting or delaying the progression to ESRD in patients with only moderately increased albuminuria (previously known as microalbuminuria or microalbumin/creatinine ratio of 30–300 mcg/mg). In patients who are normotensive, there is no evidence that use of these agents is renoprotective in the presence of albuminuria. For this reason, the ADA 2021 Standards of Medical Care for Diabetes recommend that only patients with elevated blood pressure be treated with ACEi or ARB therapy.[46] However, the Kidney Disease—Improving Global Outcomes (KDIGO) group has heavily weighted results of the SPRINT trial and recommends treatment of patients with CKD and albuminuria with ACEi or ARB therapy, with a systolic blood pressure target of less than 120 mm Hg.[47–49] Patients with albuminuria who are adequately treated to goal HbA1c, blood pressure, and low-density lipoprotein-cholesterol (LDL-C)-lowering therapy experience a nearly 50% reduction in cardiovascular and microvascular events, with an NNT of 5 after 7.8 years.[50]

ALTERNATIVE ANTIHYPERGLYCEMIC AGENTS

The CV safety and CV and renal benefits of SGLT2i, GLP1RA, and the lack of benefit of DPP4i are well characterized because these diabetes drug classes were developed after the FDA required rigorous study of the CV safety of new antihyperglycemic agents. All of the CVOTs conducted to demonstrate CV safety of antihyperglycemic drugs in type 2 diabetes were on a background of metformin therapy. Glucose-lowering agents approved before 2008 are safe, but the evidence base for ASCVD protection is less strong, without the benefit of large, randomized controlled trials with enough CV events to demonstrate these outcomes. Antihyperglycemic medications with some evidence for ASCVD benefit include metformin, acarbose, pioglitazone, and quick-release bromocriptine (Cycloset).[51] The UKPDS demonstrated a 36% relative risk reduction in all-cause mortality with metformin (NNT of 18), whereas the "Study on the Prognosis and Effect of Antidiabetic Drugs on Type 2 Diabetes Mellitus with Coronary Artery Disease" (SPREAD-DIMCAD) study of patients with type 2 diabetes and previous coronary artery disease (CAD) demonstrated a remarkable 12% absolute risk reduction in MACE (with an NNT of 8).[52,53] The mechanism for metformin's putative cardioprotective effect has not been elucidated. One proposed mechanism is that metformin stimulation of AMP-kinase pathway may have antioxidant effects in endothelial cells and antiinflammatory effects in cardiomyocytes.[54,55] Insulin and sulfonylureas have generally not been shown to increase cardiovascular risk, although studies are mixed.[51]

There is evidence for CV protection in prediabetes with acarbose, an alpha-glucosidase inhibitor. It is inexpensive, but unfortunately may not be tolerated due to gastrointestinal side effects. The "Study to Prevent Non-Insulin-Dependent Diabetes Mellitus" (STOP-NIDDM) trial of patients with impaired glucose tolerance demonstrated a 49% relative risk reduction and 2.5% absolute risk reduction (NNT of 40 over 3.3 years) of major cardiovascular events (coronary heart disease, cardiovascular death, congestive heart failure, cerebrovascular event, and peripheral vascular disease).[56] Of the components of the primary composite endpoint, the most significant was myocardial infarction, with 91% relative risk reduction. However, a Cochrane systematic review and meta-analysis of alpha-glucosidase inhibitors including acarbose concluded that there was no effect of this class of antihyperglycemic agents on morbidity or mortality.[57] Pioglitazone is effective for secondary prevention of stroke after ischemic stroke or transient ischemic attack in patients with insulin resistance (elevated homeostasis model assessment of insulin resistance [HOMA-IR] index) as demonstrated in the Insulin Resistance Intervention after Stroke (IRIS) trial.[58] A systematic review of randomized controlled trials of pioglitazone concluded that there was a significant decrease in repeat stroke (hazard ratio [HR] 0.68) and major vascular events (HR 0.75).[59] The PROactive trial demonstrated an NNT of 48 over 3 years to prevent a first cardiac event with pioglitazone therapy in type 2 diabetes.[60] Although there was initial concern for increased CV risk with rosiglitazone, the RECORD trial did not confirm these findings,[61] and the FDA subsequently lifted the black box warning for rosiglitazone but its use remains low. The thiazolidinediones should be avoided in patients with symptomatic heart failure.[62]

Bromocriptine (Cycloset) is a dopamine agonist used for prolactinoma and Parkinson disease and approved for use in type 2 diabetes. Its use is not widespread due to its high cost and side effects; however, bromocriptine use led to an absolute risk reduction of 1.4% in cardiac events, with an NNT of 71.[63]

CHOLESTEROL MANAGEMENT

Cholesterol screening when younger than 40 years may reasonably be performed every 5 years, after which time annual lipid panels should be performed. Patients with diabetes age 40 years and greater without ASCVD should be placed on statin therapy (at least moderate intensity), and the American Heart Association/American College of Cardiology Foundation ASCVD risk score should be used to assess whether statin therapy should be intensified to "high intensity" (**Table 2**). The importance of statin therapy in patients with diabetes cannot be overemphasized. A lipid panel should be drawn 4 to 12 weeks after cholesterol therapy is changed to assess compliance and effectiveness of treatment.[23] In the presence of insulin resistance and diabetes, more cholesterol is transferred to very LDL (VLDL) from LDL, leading to small dense LDL, which confers greater CV risk. In addition, hyperglycemia and glycemic variability worsen endothelial dysfunction and inflammation.[64,65] Even when LDL-C levels are not elevated, patients may be at significantly increased risk for CVD.[66]

Areas of uncertainty regarding when to initiate statin therapy exist, particularly in patients with type 1 diabetes and younger patients with type 2 diabetes. Special lipid testing is available, including apolipoprotein B (ApoB), high-sensitivity C-reactive protein (hsCRP), and lipoprotein (a) [Lp(a)] when there is uncertainty over whether a statin should be started. The American Diabetes Association (ADA) and American Heart Association (AHA) do not recommend routinely assessing Apo B because there is robust evidence for the utility of LDL-C. The 2013 AHA/ACCF guidelines for CV risk reduction and cholesterol management did away with LDL-C treatment goals, as lipid-lowering trials were predicated on intensity of statin therapy,[67] but subsequent revisions have softened this stance.

Apo-B 100 is an apolipoprotein located on atherogenic lipoproteins: VLDL, intermediate-density lipoproteins, and LDL. Unlike LDL-C, the ApoB level reflects the actual number of atherogenic particles as opposed to the amount of cholesterol in the particles as measured by VLDL-C, HDL-C, and LDL-C. In the insulin-resistant state, there may be discordance between LDL-C and ApoB levels,[68–70] especially as triglyceride (TG) levels increase to greater than 200 mg/dL. Both the American Association of Clinical Endocrinology (AACE) and the National Lipid Association (NLA)

Table 2
Statin therapy—dosing for intensity of low-density lipoprotein lowering

LDL-C Lowering[a]	High Intensity ≥50%		Moderate Intensity 30%–49%	
	Agent	Dose (mg, QD)	Agent	Dose
Statins	Atorvastatin	(40[b]) 80	Atorvastatin	10 (20)
	Rosuvastatin	20 (40)	Rosuvastatin	(5) 10
			Simvastatin	20–40[c]
			Pravastatin	40 (80)
			Lovastatin	40 (80)
			Fluvastatin	XL 80 mg 40 mg BID
			Pitavastatin	1–4

Keep in mind that individual response may vary from what was observed in the clinical trials.

Agents and doses in **boldface** were shown to reduce major CV events in randomized controlled trials (RCTs) and the Cholesterol Treatment Trialists 2010 meta-analysis.[76]

[a] LDL-C lowering that should occur with the dosage listed below each intensity.

[b] Evidence from 1 RCT only: down titration if unable to tolerate atorvastatin 80 mg in the IDEAL (Incremental Decrease through Aggressive Lipid Lowering) study. [S3.2.1-3].

[c] Although simvastatin, 80 mg, was evaluated in RCTs, initiation of simvastatin, 80 mg, or titration to 80 mg is not recommended by the FDA because of the increased risk of myopathy, including rhabdomyolysis.

Adapted from Grundy SM, Stone NJ, Bailey AL, et al. 2018 AHA/ACC/AACVPR/AAPA/ABC/ACPM/ ADA/AGS/APhA/ASPC/NLA/PCNA Guideline on the Management of Blood Cholesterol: Executive Summary: A Report of the American College of Cardiology/American Heart Association Task Force on Clinical Practice Guidelines [published correction appears in Circulation. 2019 Jun 18;139(25):e1178-e1181]. Reprinted with permission Circulation.2018;139:e1082–e1143 ©2018 American Heart Association, Inc.

recommend an ApoB target of less than 90 mg/dL for most patients with diabetes without other significant risk factors or ASCVD if a level is available.[71,72]

Lp(a) is an independent risk factor for ASCVD,[73] but there are limited data for clinical outcomes associated with Lp(a) in patients with diabetes. There is also a paucity of data regarding optimal Lp(a) threshold in diabetes, although elevated risk is seen with levels greater than 50 mg/dL in the general population.[74] Levels of Lp(a) are mainly genetically determined, and lifestyle interventions and most cholesterol-lowering medications including statins have minimal to no effect to reduce Lp(a) values.[73] Therefore, if found to be elevated, the main focus of therapy is to optimize or use more aggressive targets for other CV risk factors including LDL-C. Although there are no diabetes-specific guidelines, the NLA recommends considering measurement of Lp(a) in anyone with a first-degree relative with premature ASCVD; patients with premature ASCVD without significant identifiable risk factors at the time of the event, calcified aortic stenosis, and inadequate drop in LDL-C despite adherence to statin therapy; and patients with severe hyperlipidemia (LDL-C >190 mg/dL).[74] Once screened, the Lp(a) value does not need to be rechecked, as it is unlikely to change significantly. As with any test, it should only be drawn if the results are likely to change clinical management.

Atherosclerosis is a chronic inflammatory condition, and for this reason, there has been increased interest in antiinflammatory medications for cardiovascular protection. Diabetes is also an inflammatory condition that may contribute to the increased risk in

CVD. hsCRP is the marker with the most robust data for predicting cardiovascular events. In one large prospective study with patients with type 2 diabetes, it was found that an hsCRP greater than 3 mg/L had an HR of 1.72 for coronary heart disease after 7 years of follow-up.[75] In summary, ApoB, Lp(a), and hsCRP may be helpful in risk stratifying patients for initiation or intensification of cardiovascular protective agents in the right patients.

CHOLESTEROL MANAGEMENT—PRIMARY PREVENTION

All patients older than 40 years with type 2 diabetes and LDL-C greater than 70 mg/dL should be started on a moderate- or high-intensity statin for primary prevention based on the most recent AHA guidelines for CV risk reduction. High-intensity statins should be considered for those older than 50 years with additional CV risk factors,[23,77] based on overwhelming evidence for CV protection with statin therapy. Refer to **Box 1** for characteristics that increase CV risk independent of diabetes. Diabetes has been referred to as a cardiac risk equivalent because of the 2- to 4-fold increase in CV risk as compared with the general population, comparable with individuals with a prior ASCVD event.[78] The NLA does not recommend assessment of coronary artery calcium scores for patients with diabetes to determine which patients do not need statin therapy.[79] All of the currently commercially available statins are also available in generic form, which may help to reduce cost as a barrier for patients.

In younger patients between the ages of 20 and 40 years, it may be reasonable to start statin therapy when significant risk factors are present.[23] Clinicians should always discuss avoiding statin therapy in pregnancy and recommend appropriate contraception for women during childbearing years.[80] Although the data are not as clear for patients with type 1 diabetes, in 2020, the Endocrine Society became the first organization to release guidelines recommending statin therapy in all patients with diabetes older than 40 years and patients with type 1 diabetes with microvascular complications or duration of type 1 diabetes for more than 20 years.[81]

Box 1
Characteristics that increase cardiovascular risk in diabetes independent of other risk factors

- Long duration of diabetes
  - 10 years or greater for type 2 diabetes
- 20 years or greater for type 1 diabetes
- Albuminuria (urine ACR ≥ 30 mg albumin/g creatinine)
- Estimated GFR less than 60 mL/min/1.73 m^2
- Retinopathy
- Neuropathy
- Ankle-brachial index less than 0.9
- Lp(a) > 50
- Elevated ApoB level
- hs-CRP greater than 3
- Unhealthy diet
- Inactivity—including prolonged sedentary time

Abbreviations: ACR, albumin-to-creatinine ratio; GFR, glomerular filtration rate.

A good rule of thumb is that every 40 mg/dL drop in LDL-C results in an approximately 20% reduction in CV events and 10% reduction in mortality.[82] Collaborative Atorvastatin Diabetes Study (CARDS) was a randomized controlled trial of 2838 patients with diabetes between the ages of 40 and 75 years demonstrating that treating 1000 people with atorvastatin, 10 mg, for 4 years would prevent 37 major cardiac events (NNT of 31).[83] Moderate-intensity statins are defined as dosing that results in a 30% to 49% decline in LDL-C levels, whereas high-intensity statins result in an LDL-C decrease of 50% or more. Although current cholesterol management guidelines do not target specific LDL-C levels for primary prevention, additional therapy may be added if patients have additional risk factors or do not achieve the expected effect on LDL-C after confirmation of compliance.[23] The recommended second-line agent is ezetimibe, which has been shown to provide additional CV protection following a recent CV event when added to a statin (NNT of 50 over a 6-year period).[23,84] The ACCORD Lipid trial did not show additional benefit when fenofibrate was added to statin therapy.[85] Lastly, colesevelam has an indication for HbA1c lowering, and also lowers LDL-C, but has less robust data for CV risk reduction and may be less well tolerated than ezetimibe. Furthermore, it can worsen hypertriglyceridemia and should be avoided in patients with TGs greater than 300 mg/dL.[86,87]

CHOLESTEROL MANAGEMENT—SECONDARY PREVENTION

All patients with known ASCVD with or without diabetes should be on high-intensity statin therapy with a goal LDL-C of less than 70 mg/dL.[23] In fact, following percutaneous coronary intervention for an acute coronary syndrome, no benefit of lipid-lowering therapy is manifest unless LDL-C of less than 70 mg/dL is achieved within 1 year.[88] Additional therapies including ezetimibe and PCSK-9 inhibitors should be used as needed to achieve these LDL-C targets. PCSK-9 inhibitors are costly, but are generally well tolerated and very effective at lowering LDL-C, and have been demonstrated to reduce CV risk.[23]

TRIGLYCERIDE LOWERING

Hypertriglyceridemia should be treated when the TG concentration is greater than 500 mg/dL to lower the risk of pancreatitis. Because uncontrolled diabetes leads to decreased lipoprotein lipase (LPL) activity, and LPL is needed to clear TGs, TG concentrations greater than 500 mg/dL are not uncommon in diabetes. In addition to weight loss, consuming a diet lower in saturated fat and higher in complex carbohydrates, avoiding alcohol intake, and improving glycemic control, the use of high-dose omega-3 fatty acids and fenofibrate are preferred to reduce TG levels. Fenofibrate does not seem to carry the same risk for rhabdomyolysis as gemfibrozil and has a good safety profile even when used in conjunction with statins. Although elevated TG is associated with CV disease, lowering TG has not consistently been shown to reduce risk of CVD.[23] The REDUCE-IT trial demonstrated that in patients with established CVD or diabetes and other risk factors, TG 135 to 499 mg/dL and LDL-C 41 to 100 mg/dL, the use of icosapent ethyl, a purified omega-3 fatty acid, reduced CV events by 25% (NNT of 21 after approximately 5 years), likely through a TG-independent mechanism.[89]

BLOOD PRESSURE CONTROL

Blood pressure control is an often-overlooked major CV risk factor that in most patients is also the easiest to control. When albuminuria is not present, any of the JNC-8 preferred agents may be started without preference.[23,90] If thiazides are used, the ADA recommends use of chlorthalidone or indapamide, which have been demonstrated to decrease CV risk.[91] Targets for blood pressure control vary based on the guideline, but the ADA generally recommends targeting less than 140/90 mm Hg in lower-risk patients and less than 130/80 mm Hg in those with ASCVD, CKD, or ASCVD 10-year risk of greater than 15%.[23] The ACCORD blood pressure study did not show additional benefit of more intensive blood pressure targets in patients with diabetes.[91]

When blood pressure is initially found to be greater than 160/100 mm Hg, the patient should be started immediately on dual blood pressure medication therapy.[23] Simultaneous use of an ACEi and an ARB should be avoided, as this was shown to result in more harm without additional benefit.[92]

Clinicians should consider using combination pills in order to reduce pill burden, as diabetes is a chronic disease that often requires many daily medications, which can be discouraging to patients and lead to diabetes-related stress and/or depression. The AHA and KDIGO support the use of multiple blood pressure measurements when taken in the office similar to what was done during the SPRINT trial.[47,49] Home blood pressure measurements and ambulatory blood pressure monitoring have been shown to be superior to those measured in the clinic but may lead to delays in treatment.[93,94]

ANTIPLATELET AND ANTITHROMBOTIC THERAPY

Last but not the least to consider in addressing cardiovascular protection for patients with diabetes are antiplatelet and antithrombotic agents. Low-dose aspirin therapy for primary prevention has long been debated and is still controversial in patients with diabetes. The ADA does not recommend aspirin for primary prevention in most patients with diabetes but states that it should be considered in patients between the ages of 50 and 70 years with at least one additional major cardiovascular risk factor.[23] In those considering aspirin therapy, coronary artery calcium (CAC) scores may be helpful—patients with CAC score greater than 100 benefit from aspirin therapy.[95,96] A Study of Cardiovascular Events in Diabetes (ASCEND) demonstrated a 1.1% absolute risk reduction (NNT of 91) in major cardiac events with a 0.9% absolute increase in major bleeding events in patients with diabetes under fairly good glycemic control (HbA1c generally <8%) over a 7.4-year period.[97]

For secondary prevention, there is a strong evidence base for aspirin and/or clopidogrel in preventing ASCVD events. These agents along with statin therapy should be assessed regularly for compliance in those with known ASCVD, as they are crucial in secondary prevention.[23] Recently, the Cardiovascular Outcomes for People Using Anticoagulation Strategies (COMPASS) trial demonstrated that low-dose rivaroxaban, 2.5 mg, PO BID in addition to low-dose aspirin reduces the risk of limb amputation and major adverse cardiac events in patients with stable peripheral artery disease and/or stable CAD.[98] In addition, the Vascular Outcomes Study of ASA Along With Rivaroxaban in Endovascular or Surgical Limb Revascularization for Peripheral Artery Disease (VOYAGER PAD) trial recently demonstrated significant reduction in risk of major adverse limb or cardiac events in patients who started low-dose rivaroxaban therapy and low-dose aspirin (clopidogrel was used at the treating physicians' discretion) immediately after lower extremity revascularization without a significant increase in bleeding risk.[99]

SUMMARY

Patients with diabetes are at very high risk for atherosclerotic cardiovascular disease and mortality. Strong evidence supports aggressive management of CV risk factors to reduce risk of cardiovascular complications. The past decade has brought remarkable advances in medication therapy to lower CVD risk, including strong evidence for CV risk reduction with new antihyperglycemic drug classes (GLP1RA and SGLT2i), icosapent ethyl, PCSK9i, and an antithrombotic agent (rivaroxaban), leading to significant changes in guidelines for glycemic control, blood pressure, cholesterol-lowering, and antithrombotic therapy and renewed hope for improving macrovascular disease outcomes further in patients with diabetes.

CLINICS CARE POINTS

Primary Care Clinics—Macrovascular Complications Care Points
- Metformin is the first-line medication for type 2 diabetes.
- If a patient with type 2 diabetes has known ASCVD, heart failure, and/or CKD, a GLP1RA or SGLT2i with proven cardiovascular benefit should be initiated even if the patient's HbA1c is at goal.
- For category A2 urine albumin-to-creatinine ratio elevation (30–300 mg/g), an ACEi or ARB is indicated in the setting of elevated blood pressure.
- SGLT2i should be started when albumin-to-creatinine ratio is elevated regardless of blood pressure.
- A more intensive blood pressure goal (<130/80 mm Hg) should be targeted when patients have additional CV risk.
- A moderate- or high-intensity statin is recommended for patients with diabetes aged 40 years and older.
- Ezetimibe or PCSK9i should be added if additional LDL-C lowering is needed in patients with high CV risk.
- Icosapent ethyl and rivaroxaban, 2.5 mg, plus low-dose aspirin (81–100 mg) daily should be considered in those with or at high risk for ASCVD.

DISCLOSURE

The authors have nothing to disclose.

REFERENCES

1. American Diabetes Association. Economic costs of diabetes in the U.S. in 2017. Diabetes Care 2018;41:917–28.
2. Booth GL, Kapral MK, Fung K, et al. Relation between age and cardiovascular disease in men and women with diabetes compared with non-diabetic people: a population-based retrospective cohort study. Lancet 2006;368(9529):29–36.
3. Tancredi M, Rosengren A, Svensson AM, et al. Excess Mortality among Persons with Type 2 Diabetes. N Engl J Med 2015;373:1720–32.
4. Deshpande AD, Harris-Hayes M, Schootman M. Epidemiology of diabetes and diabetes-related complications. Phys Ther 2008;88(11):1254–64.
5. Gregg EW, Li Y, Wang J, et al. Changes in diabetes-related complications in the United States, 1990-2010. N Engl J Med 2014;370:1514–23.
6. Ali MK, Bullard KM, Saaddine JB, et al. Achievement of goals in U.S. diabetes care, 1999-2010. N Engl J Med 2013;368:1613–24.
7. Bax JJ, Young LH, Frye RL, et al. Screening for coronary artery disease in patients with diabetes. Diabetes Care 2007;30:2729–36.
8. Young LH, Wackers FJT, Chyun DA, et al. DIAD Investigators. Cardiac outcomes after screening for asymptomatic coronary artery disease in patients with type 2 diabetes: the DIAD study: a randomized controlled trial. JAMA 2009;301: 1547–55.

9. Franz MJ, Boucher JL, Rutten-Ramos S, et al. Lifestyle weight-loss intervention outcomes in overweight and obese adults with type 2 diabetes: a systemic review and meta-analysis of randomized controlled trials. J Acad Nutr Diet 2015;115: 1447–63.

10. American Diabetes Association. 8. Obesity management for the treatment of Type 2 diabetes: standards of medical care in diabetes—2021. Diabetes Care 2021;44(Suppl 1):S100–10.

11. Lean ME, Leslie WS, Barnes AC, et al. Primary care-led weight management for remission of type 2 diabetes (DiRECT): an open-label, cluster-randomised trial. Lancet 2018;391(10120):541–51.

12. Kodama S, Tanaka S, Heianza Y, et al. Association between physical activity and risk of all-cause mortality and cardiovascular disease in patients with diabetes: a meta-analysis. Diabetes Care 2013;36(2):471–9.

13. Rubino F, Nathan DM, Eckel RH, et al. Delegates of the 2nd diabetes surgery summit. metabolic surgery in the treatment algorithm for type 2 diabetes: a joint statement by international diabetes organizations. Diabetes Care 2016;39:861–77.

14. O'Brien R, Johnson E, Haneuse S, et al. Microvascular outcomes in patients with diabetes after bariatric surgery versus usual care: A Matched Cohort Study. Ann Intern Med 2018;169(5):300–10.

15. Schauer PR, Bhatt DL, Kirwan JP, et al. Bariatric surgery versus intensive medical therapy for diabetes–3-year outcomes. N Engl J Med 2014;370(21):2002–13.

16. Bramante CT, Raatz S, Bomberg EM, et al. Cardiovascular risks and benefits of medications used for weight loss. Front Endocrinol (Lausanne) 2020;10:883.

17. Stratton IM, Adler AI, Neil HA, et al. Association of glycaemia with macrovascular and microvascular complications of type 2 diabetes (UKPDS 35): prospective observational study. BMJ 2000;321(7258):405–12.

18. Holman RR, Paul SK, Bethel MA, et al. 10-year follow-up of intensive glucose control in type 2 diabetes. N Engl J Med 2008;359(15):1577–89.

19. Nathan DM, Cleary PA, Backlund JY, et al. Intensive diabetes treatment and cardiovascular disease in patients with type 1 diabetes. N Engl J Med 2005;353(25): 2643–53.

20. Intensive blood-glucose control with sulphonylureas or insulin compared with conventional treatment and risk of complications in patients with type 2 diabetes (UKPDS 33). UK Prospective Diabetes Study (UKPDS) Group. Lancet 1998; 352(9131):837–53 [Erratum appears in Lancet 1999;354(9178):602.

21. Chalmers J, Cooper ME. UKPDS and the legacy effect. N Engl J Med 2008;359: 1618–20.

22. American Diabetes Association. 9. Pharmacologic Approaches to Glycemic Treatment: Standards of Medical Care in Diabetes—2021. Diabetes Care 2021; 44(Suppl 1):S111–24.

23. American Diabetes Association. 10. Cardiovascular Disease and Risk Management: Standards of Medical Care in Diabetes—2021. Diabetes Care 2021; 44(Suppl 1):S125–50.

24. Cosmi F, Laini R, Nicolucci A. Semaglutide and cardiovascular outcomes in patients with Type 2 diabetes. N Engl J Med 2017;376(9):890.

25. Marso SP, Daniels GH, Brown-Frandsen K, et al. Liraglutide and cardiovascular outcomes in Type 2 diabetes. N Engl J Med 2016;375(4):311–22.

26. Del Olmo-Garcia MI, Merino-Torres JF. GLP-1 receptor agonists and cardiovascular disease in patients with Type 2 diabetes. J Diabetes Res 2018;2018:4020492.

27. Zinman B, Lachin JM, Inzucchi SE. Empagliflozin, cardiovascular outcomes, and mortality in Type 2 diabetes. N Engl J Med 2016;374(11):1094.

28. Anderson SL, Marrs JC. Antihyperglycemic medications and cardiovascular risk reduction. Eur Endocrinol 2017;13(2):86–90.
29. Neal B, Perkovic V, Matthews DR. Canagliflozin and cardiovascular and renal events in Type 2 diabetes. N Engl J Med 2017;377(21):2099.
30. Wiviott SD, Raz I, Bonaca MP, et al. Dapagliflozin and cardiovascular outcomes in Type 2 diabetes. N Engl J Med 2019;380(4):347–57.
31. Silverii GA, Monami M, Mannucci E. Sodium-glucose co-transporter-2 inhibitors and all-cause mortality: a meta-analysis of randomized controlled trials. Diabetes Obes Metab 2021;23(4):1052–6.
32. Cannon CP, Pratley R, Dagogo-Jack S, et al. Cardiovascular outcomes with ertugliflozin in Type 2 diabetes. N Engl J Med 2020;383(15):1425–35.
33. Zelniker TA, Wiviott SD, Raz I, et al. Comparison of the effects of glucagon-like peptide receptor agonists and sodium-glucose cotransporter 2 inhibitors for prevention of major adverse cardiovascular and renal outcomes in Type 2 diabetes mellitus. Circulation 2019;139(17):2022–31.
34. Zelniker TA, Wiviott SD, Raz I, et al. SGLT2 inhibitors for primary and secondary prevention of cardiovascular and renal outcomes in type 2 diabetes: a systematic review and meta-analysis of cardiovascular outcome trials. Lancet 2019; 393(10166):31–9 [Erratum appears in Lancet 2019;393(10166):30].
35. Gerstein HC, Colhoun HM, Dagenais GR, et al. Dulaglutide and cardiovascular outcomes in type 2 diabetes (REWIND): a double-blind, randomised placebo-controlled trial. Lancet 2019;394(10193):121–30.
36. McMurray JJV, Solomon SD, Inzucchi SE, et al. Dapagliflozin in patients with heart failure and reduced ejection fraction. N Engl J Med 2019;381(21):1995–2008.
37. Packer M, Anker SD, Butler J, et al. Empagliflozin in patients with heart failure, reduced ejection fraction, and volume overload: EMPEROR-Reduced Trial. J Am Coll Cardiol 2021;77(11):1381–92.
38. Packer M. Do DPP-4 inhibitors cause heart failure events by promoting adrenergically mediated cardiotoxicity? Clues from laboratory models and clinical trials. Circ Res 2018;122(7):928–32.
39. Heerspink HJL, Stefánsson BV, Correa-Rotter R, et al. Dapagliflozin in patients with chronic kidney disease. N Engl J Med 2020;383(15):1436–46.
40. Perkovic V, Jardine MJ, Neal B, et al. Canagliflozin and renal outcomes in Type 2 diabetes and nephropathy. N Engl J Med 2019;380(24):2295–306.
41. Lewis EJ, Hunsicker LG, Bain RP, et al. The effect of angiotensin-converting-enzyme inhibition on diabetic nephropathy. The Collaborative Study Group. N Engl J Med 1993;329(20):1456–62 [Erratum appears in N Engl J Med 1993;330(2):152].
42. Brenner BM, Cooper ME, de Zeeuw D, et al. Effects of losartan on renal and cardiovascular outcomes in patients with type 2 diabetes and nephropathy. N Engl J Med 2001;345(12):861–9.
43. Lewis EJ, Hunsicker LG, Clarke WR, et al. Renoprotective effect of the angiotensin-receptor antagonist irbesartan in patients with nephropathy due to type 2 diabetes. N Engl J Med 2001;345(12):851–60.
44. Mauer M, Zinman B, Gardiner R, et al. Renal and retinal effects of enalapril and losartan in type 1 diabetes. N Engl J Med 2009;361(1):40–51.
45. Weil EJ, Fufaa G, Jones LI, et al. Erratum. Effect of losartan on prevention and progression of early diabetic nephropathy in American Indians With Type 2 Diabetes. Diabetes 2013;62:3224-3231. Diabetes 2018;67(3):532.

46. American Diabetes Association. 11. Microvascular Complications and Foot Care: Standards of Medical Care in Diabetes-2021. Diabetes Care 2021; 44(Suppl 1):S151–67.

47. Cheung AK, Chang TI, Cushman WC, et al. Executive summary of the KDIGO 2021 clinical practice guideline for the management of blood pressure in Chronic Kidney Disease. Kidney Int 2021;99(3):559–69.

48. Cheung AK, Rahman M, Reboussin DM, et al. Effects of intensive BP control in CKD. J Am Soc Nephrol 2017;28(9):2812–23.

49. SPRINT Research Group, Wright JT Jr, Williamson JD, et al. A randomized trial of intensive versus standard blood-pressure control. N Engl J Med 2015;373(22): 2103–16 [Erratum appears in N Engl J Med 2017;377(25):2506].

50. Gaede P, Vedel P, Larsen N, et al. Multifactorial intervention and cardiovascular disease in patients with type 2 diabetes. N Engl J Med 2003;348(5):383–93.

51. Low Wang CC, Hess CN, Hiatt WR, et al. Clinical update: cardiovascular disease in diabetes mellitus: atherosclerotic cardiovascular disease and heart failure in Type 2 diabetes mellitus - mechanisms, management, and clinical considerations. Circulation 2016;133(24):2459–502.

52. Effect of intensive blood-glucose control with metformin on complications in overweight patients with type 2 diabetes (UKPDS 34). UK Prospective Diabetes Study (UKPDS) Group. Lancet 1998;352(9131):854–65 [Erratum appears in Lancet 1998;352(9139):1558].

53. Hong J, Zhang Y, Lai S, et al. Effects of metformin versus glipizide on cardiovascular outcomes in patients with type 2 diabetes and coronary artery disease. Diabetes Care 2013;36(5):1304–11.

54. Giaccari A, Solini A, Frontoni S, et al. Metformin benefits: another example for alternative energy substrate mechanism? Diabetes Care 2021;44(3):647–54.

55. Sambe T, Mason RP, Dawoud H, et al. Metformin treatment decreases nitroxidative stress, restores nitric oxide bioavailability and endothelial function beyond glucose control. Biomed Pharmacother 2018;98:149–56.

56. Chiasson JL, Josse RG, Gomis R, et al. Acarbose treatment and the risk of cardiovascular disease and hypertension in patients with impaired glucose tolerance: the STOP-NIDDM trial. JAMA 2003;290(4):486–94.

57. van de Laar FA, Lucassen PL, Akkermans RP, et al. Alpha-glucosidase inhibitors for patients with type 2 diabetes: results from a Cochrane systematic review and meta-analysis. Diabetes Care 2005;28(1):154–63.

58. Kernan WN, Viscoli CM, Furie KL, et al. Pioglitazone after ischemic stroke or transient ischemic attack. N Engl J Med 2016;374(14):1321–31.

59. Lee M, Saver JL, Liao HW, et al. Pioglitazone for secondary stroke prevention: a systematic review and meta-analysis. Stroke 2017;48(2):388–93.

60. Dormandy JA, Charbonnel B, Eckland DJ, et al. Secondary prevention of macrovascular events in patients with type 2 diabetes in the PROactive Study (PROspective pioglitAzone Clinical Trial In macroVascular Events): a randomised controlled trial. Lancet 2005;366(9493):1279–89.

61. Home PD, Pocock SJ, Beck-Nielsen H, et al. Rosiglitazone evaluated for cardiovascular outcomes in oral agent combination therapy for type 2 diabetes (RECORD): a multicentre, randomised, open-label trial. Lancet 2009;373(9681): 2125–35.

62. Nesto RW, Bell D, Bonow RO, et al. Thiazolidinedione use, fluid retention, and congestive heart failure: a consensus statement from the American Heart Association and American Diabetes Association. Diabetes Care 2004;27(1):256–63.

63. Gaziano JM, Cincotta AH, O'Connor CM, et al. Erratum. Randomized clinical trial of quick-release bromocriptine among patients with Type 2 diabetes on overall safety and cardiovascular outcomes. Diabetes Care 2016;39(10):1846.

64. Ceriello A, Kilpatrick ES. Glycemic variability: both sides of the story. Diabetes Care 2013;36(Suppl 2):S272–5.

65. Krauss RM. Lipids and lipoproteins in patients with type 2 diabetes. Diabetes Care 2004;27(6):1496–504.

66. Haffner SM, Lehto S, Rönnemaa T, et al. Mortality from coronary heart disease in subjects with type 2 diabetes and in nondiabetic subjects with and without prior myocardial infarction. N Engl J Med 1998;339(4):229–34.

67. Stone NJ, Robinson JG, Lichtenstein AH, et al. 2013 ACC/AHA guideline on the treatment of blood cholesterol to reduce atherosclerotic cardiovascular risk in adults: a report of the American College of Cardiology/American Heart Association Task Force on Practice Guidelines. J Am Coll Cardiol 2014;63(25 Pt B): 2889–934 [Erratum appears in J Am Coll Cardiol 2014;63(25 Pt B):3024-3025; Erratum appears in J Am Coll Cardiol 2015;66(24):2812].

68. Sniderman A, Langlois M, Cobbaert C. Update on apolipoprotein B. Curr Opin Lipidol 2021. https://doi.org/10.1097/MOL.0000000000000754 [published online ahead of print, 2021].

69. Wilkins JT, Li RC, Sniderman A, et al. Discordance between apolipoprotein B and LDL-cholesterol in young adults predicts coronary artery calcification: The CARDIA Study. J Am Coll Cardiol 2016;67(2):193–201.

70. Rabizadeh S, Rajab A, Mechanick JI, et al. LDL/apo B ratio predict coronary heart disease in Type 2 diabetes independent of ASCVD risk score: a case-cohort study. Nutr Metab Cardiovasc Dis 2021;31(5):1477–85.

71. Jacobson TA, Ito MK, Maki KC, et al. National Lipid Association recommendations for patient-centered management of dyslipidemia: part 1–full report. J Clin Lipidol 2015;9(2):129–69.

72. Jellinger PS. American Association of Clinical Endocrinologists/American College of Endocrinology Management of Dyslipidemia and Prevention of Cardiovascular Disease Clinical Practice Guidelines. Diabetes Spectr 2018;31(3):234–45.

73. McCormick SP. Lipoprotein(a): biology and clinical importance. Clin Biochem Rev 2004;25(1):69–80.

74. Wilson DP, Jacobson TA, Jones PH, et al. Use of Lipoprotein(a) in clinical practice: a biomarker whose time has come. A scientific statement from the National Lipid Association. J Clin Lipidol 2019;13(3):374–92.

75. Soinio M, Marniemi J, Laakso M, et al. High-sensitivity C-reactive protein and coronary heart disease mortality in patients with type 2 diabetes: a 7-year follow-up study. Diabetes Care 2006;29(2):329–33.

76. Cholesterol Treatment Trialists' (CTT) Collaboration, Baigent C, Blackwell L, et al. Efficacy and safety of more intensive lowering of LDL cholesterol: a meta-analysis of data from 170,000 participants in 26 randomised trials. Lancet 2010; 376(9753):1670–81.

77. Grundy SM, Stone NJ, Bailey AL, et al. 2018 AHA/ACC/AACVPR/AAPA/ABC/ ACPM/ADA/AGS/APhA/ASPC/NLA/PCNA Guideline on the Management of Blood Cholesterol: Executive Summary: A Report of the American College of Cardiology/American Heart Association Task Force on Clinical Practice Guidelines. Circulation 2019;139(25):e1046–81 [Erratum appears in Circulation 2019;139(25): e1178-e1181].

78. Emerging Risk Factors Collaboration, Sarwar N, Gao P, et al. Diabetes mellitus, fasting blood glucose concentration, and risk of vascular disease: a collaborative

meta-analysis of 102 prospective studies. Lancet 2010;375(9733):2215–22 [Erratum appears in Lancet. 2010;376(9745):958. Hillage, H L [corrected to Hillege, H L]].

79. Orringer CE, Blaha MJ, Blankstein R, et al. The National Lipid Association scientific statement on coronary artery calcium scoring to guide preventive strategies for ASCVD risk reduction. J Clin Lipidol 2021;15(1):33–60.

80. American Diabetes Association. Diabetes Care 2021;44(Suppl 1):S180–99.

81. Newman CB, Blaha MJ, Boord JB, et al. Lipid Management in Patients with Endocrine Disorders: An Endocrine Society Clinical Practice Guideline. J Clin Endocrinol Metab 2020;105(12):dgaa674 [Erratum appears in J Clin Endocrinol Metab 2021;106(6):e2465].

82. Cholesterol Treatment Trialists' (CTT) Collaborators, Kearney PM, Blackwell L, et al. Efficacy of cholesterol-lowering therapy in 18,686 people with diabetes in 14 randomised trials of statins: a meta-analysis. Lancet 2008;371(9607):117–25.

83. Colhoun HM, Betteridge DJ, Durrington PN, et al. Primary prevention of cardiovascular disease with atorvastatin in type 2 diabetes in the Collaborative Atorvastatin Diabetes Study (CARDS): multicentre randomised placebo-controlled trial. Lancet 2004;364(9435):685–96.

84. Cannon CP, Blazing MA, Giugliano RP, et al. Ezetimibe Added to Statin Therapy after Acute Coronary Syndromes. N Engl J Med 2015;372(25):2387–97.

85. ACCORD Study Group, Ginsberg HN, Elam MB, et al. Effects of combination lipid therapy in type 2 diabetes mellitus. N Engl J Med 2010;362(17):1563–74 [Erratum appears in N Engl J Med 2010;362(18):1748].

86. Schwab P, Louder A, Li Y, et al. Cholesterol treatment patterns and cardiovascular clinical outcomes associated with colesevelam HCl and ezetimibe. Drugs Aging 2014;31(9):683–94.

87. Bays H, Jones PH. Colesevelam hydrochloride: reducing atherosclerotic coronary heart disease risk factors. Vasc Health Risk Manag 2007;3(5):733–42.

88. Farkouh ME, Godoy LC, Brooks MM, et al. Influence of LDL-cholesterol lowering on cardiovascular outcomes in patients with diabetes mellitus undergoing coronary revascularization. J Am Coll Cardiol 2020;76(19):2197–207.

89. Bhatt DL, Steg PG, Miller M, et al. Cardiovascular risk reduction with icosapent ethyl for hypertriglyceridemia. N Engl J Med 2019;380(1):11–22.

90. James PA, Oparil S, Carter BL, et al. 2014 evidence-based guideline for the management of high blood pressure in adults: report from the panel members appointed to the Eighth Joint National Committee (JNC 8). JAMA 2014;311(5):507–20 [Erratum appears in JAMA 2014;311(17):1809].

91. ACCORD Study Group, Cushman WC, Evans GW, et al. Effects of intensive blood-pressure control in type 2 diabetes mellitus. N Engl J Med 2010;362(17):1575–85.

92. ONTARGET Investigators, Yusuf S, Teo KK, et al. Telmisartan, ramipril, or both in patients at high risk for vascular events. N Engl J Med 2008;358(15):1547–59.

93. Bobrie G, Genès N, Vaur L, et al. Is "isolated home" hypertension as opposed to "isolated office" hypertension a sign of greater cardiovascular risk? Arch Intern Med 2001;161(18):2205–11.

94. Sega R, Facchetti R, Bombelli M, et al. Prognostic value of ambulatory and home blood pressures compared with office blood pressure in the general population: follow-up results from the Pressioni Arteriose Monitorate e Loro Associazioni (PAMELA) study. Circulation 2005;111(14):1777–83.

95. Cainzos-Achirica M, Miedema MD, McEvoy JW, et al. Coronary artery calcium for personalized allocation of aspirin in primary prevention of Cardiovascular

Disease in 2019: The MESA Study (Multi-Ethnic Study of Atherosclerosis). Circulation 2020;141(19):1541–53.

96. Mortensen MB, Dzaye O, Steffensen FH, et al. Impact of plaque burden versus stenosis on ischemic events in patients with coronary atherosclerosis. J Am Coll Cardiol 2020;76(24):2803–13.

97. Bowman L, Mafham M, Stevens W, et al. ASCEND: A Study of Cardiovascular Events iN Diabetes: characteristics of a randomized trial of aspirin and of omega-3 fatty acid supplementation in 15,480 people with diabetes. Am Heart J 2018;198:135–44.

98. Eikelboom JW, Connolly SJ, Bosch J, et al. Rivaroxaban with or without aspirin in stable cardiovascular Disease. N Engl J Med 2017;377(14):1319–30.

99. Ultee KHJ, Steunenberg SL, Schouten O. Rivaroxaban in peripheral artery disease after revascularization. N Engl J Med 2020;383(21):2089–90.

Diabetes-Associated Comorbidities

Julia Teck, MD

KEYWORDS

- Diabetes • Comorbidities • Hypertension • NAFLD • PCOS • Obesity
- Sleep apnea • Dyslipidemia

KEY POINTS

- The most common diabetes-associated conditions share a bidirectional pathogenic relationship.
- Diabetic comorbidities hypertension, dyslipidemia, fatty liver disease, PCOS, obesity, and OSA result from multifactorial pathways caused by modifiable and nonmodifiable risk factors that intersect with diabetes.
- Lifestyle interventions of diet modification, increased physical activity, and weight loss are among first-line treatments for all of these conditions.

INTRODUCTION

This article focuses on the best-known comorbid diseases associated specifically with type 2 diabetes and their comanagement. In any of these comorbidities, a patient-centered approach with an assessment of patient preferences and beliefs is recommended when determining treatment.[1]

HYPERTENSION
Prevalence

Data show that a total of 1.13 billion people worldwide have hypertension.[2] Nearly half of adults in the United States have hypertension,[3] and it is expected that only 24% of adults have well-controlled hypertension.[4]

Hypertension is estimated to be present in two-thirds of patients with diabetes.[5] Hypertension is a diabetes risk factor, and the incidence of hypertension increases notably in a population of patients with diabetes.[6]

Overview of Disease

The definition of hypertension and target blood pressures for specific patient groups vary slightly based on the guidelines selected. Most medical societies, including the

Duke/Southern Regional Area Health Education Center, 1601 Owen Drive, Fayetteville, NC 28304, USA
E-mail address: Julia.Teck@sr-ahec.org

Prim Care Clin Office Pract 49 (2022) 275–286
https://doi.org/10.1016/j.pop.2021.11.004
primarycare.theclinics.com
0095-4543/22/© 2021 Elsevier Inc. All rights reserved.

American Diabetes Association (ADA),[7] currently define hypertension as sustained blood pressure readings with systolic blood pressure greater than or equal to 140 and a diastolic blood pressure greater than or equal to 90 on at least two occurrences.[8–11] All providers must be diligent in ensuring that any patients with a first elevated blood pressure have adequate follow-up with repeat blood pressure readings.

Prompt diagnosis and management of hypertension are essential because of the multiple complications that can arise from untreated or uncontrolled hypertension.[11] Risks of cardiovascular disease (CVD), heart failure, stroke, peripheral artery disease, and abdominal aortic aneurysm each increase as systolic and/or diastolic blood pressures increase.[12]

The Relationship Between Hypertension and Diabetes

Diabetes and hypertension share several pathophysiologic mechanisms:[13,14]

- Inappropriate activation of the renin-angiotensin-aldosterone system
- Oxidative stress
- Microvascular inflammation
- Increased sympathetic nervous activation
- Impaired insulin-mediated vasodilation
- Abnormal sodium processing in the kidneys

In the development of hypertension, insulin resistance can lead to inflammatory abnormalities in the vasculature causing stiff hypertrophic vessels and vascular remodeling.[14] This leads to significantly higher CVD risk in diabetes associated with hypertension, once again illustrating the additive effect of one condition on the other.[6,14] Therefore, the ADA recommends measuring blood pressure in patients with diabetes at every routine clinical visit.[7]

Combined Treatment of Hypertension and Diabetes

The end goal of hypertension treatment in patients with or without diabetes is proper control of blood pressure values. The ADA recommends individualized blood pressure targets; at minimum hypertension in patients with diabetes should be treated to less than 140/90. In addition to the multiple options for pharmacologic treatment, diet and lifestyle changes are recommended[7]:

- Increasing activity
- Appropriate weight loss
- Sodium intake of less than 2300 mg/d
- Decreasing alcohol consumption
- Dietary Approaches to Stop Hypertension (DASH) eating plan, which is the most evidence-based diet plan

Prompt initiation of hypertension treatment is essential. The Eighth Joint National Committee (JNC 8) recommends initial hypertension treatment with a thiazide-type diuretic, calcium channel blocker, angiotensin-converting enzyme (ACE) inhibitor, or angiotensin receptor blocker (ARB) in the general non-African American adult population regardless of the presence of diabetes.[8] In the general African American hypertensive population, thiazide diuretics or calcium channel blocker are first-line. These JNC 8 recommendations are unchanged for patients with diabetes because multiple studies illustrated no difference in major cardiovascular outcomes based on treatment choice.[8] However, the ADA provides more specific guidelines and recommends an angiotensin-converting enzyme inhibitor or angiotensin receptor blocker as first-line in hypertensive patients with diabetes if they also have a preexisting history of CVD or albuminuria.[7]

OBESITY
Prevalence

Rates of obesity are quickly increasing around the globe. Obesity prevalence increased from 30.5% in 2000 to 42.4% in 2018.[15,16] Obesity rates vary according to race and socioeconomic status, highlighting the effects of health disparities on health outcomes.[1,16]

Overview of Disease

Obesity is a multifactorial health issue of excess body fat deposition that results from a combination of individual nonmodifiable risk factors and modifiable behavioral factors.[17,18] The common metric of obesity is body mass index (BMI): an individual's weight (in kilograms) divided by the square of their height (in meters squared). BMI is not a direct measurement of body fat but it correlates with other more direct measurements and is more easily calculated.[18] BMI categories are as follows[18]:

- Underweight: BMI <18.5
- Healthy weight: BMI 18.5–24.9
- Overweight: BMI 25.0–29.9
- Obesity: BMI $\geq$30

Obesity affects multiple conditions including CVD and cerebrovascular disease, diabetes, sleep apnea, certain types of cancer, and all-cause mortality.[1,16] Providers must counsel patients who are overweight or obese of their increased risk of these adverse health outcomes and develop an individualized plan to improve their lifestyle.[1]

The Relationship Between Obesity and Diabetes

Obesity is a modifiable risk factor for diabetes. Proper management of obesity can delay the progression of prediabetes to overt diabetes. Sustained weight loss in obese patients with diabetes improves glycemic control and can decrease the number of diabetic medications needed.[1]

Both obesity and diabetes are multifactorial conditions, interrelated through mechanisms that are still being examined. Most fundamentally, obesity is a known cause of insulin resistance, which contributes to the later development of diabetes.[19–21] Obese patients have increased deposition of fat in skeletal muscle tissue causing insulin resistance through interference with glucose transport and insulin signaling.[20] Recent research studies on epigenetics also reveal that specific epigenetic changes also contribute to insulin resistance in obesity.[21] Cells become more resistant to insulin with progressive increase in fatty tissue and decreased physical activity.[20]

Combined Treatment of Obesity and Diabetes

The treatment of obesity overlaps the treatment of diabetes. It is important for providers to evaluate the systemic, structural, and socioeconomic factors affecting each patient that may influence their lifestyle patterns.

Lifestyle adjustments are the cornerstone of treatment. The recommendation for all overweight and obese patients with diabetes is to achieve and sustain at least a 5% weight loss. Large-scale trials concluded that patients who underwent intensive lifestyle adjustment required fewer glucose-lowering, lipid-lowering, and antihypertensive medications.[1]

In managing obesity in patients with diabetes, providers must be aware that certain diabetic medications can have positive or negative effects on weight. In general, providers should review the patient's entire medication list for other medications that can affect weight gain.[1] For certain patients with diabetes with an overweight or obese BMI, weight loss medications are used selectively as effective adjuncts.

If lifestyle changes and weight-loss medication adjuncts are not sufficient for sustained weight loss, metabolic surgery should be considered, especially for all patients with diabetes who are surgical candidates with BMI greater than or equal to 40. Multiple randomized trials have identified several forms of gastrointestinal surgeries (vertical sleeve gastrectomy and Roux-en-Y gastric bypass) that lead to sustained weight loss and improvement in hyperglycemia.[1]

POLYCYSTIC OVARY SYNDROME
Prevalence

Polycystic ovary syndrome (PCOS) is a complex endocrinologic condition that is one of the most common causes of infertility in women,[22] and estimated to affect 6% to 12% of reproductive-age women in the United States.[23,24] Insulin resistance is frequently seen in PCOS and more than half of women with PCOS develop diabetes by the age of 40.[23]

Overview of Disease

PCOS pathogenesis understanding is fairly limited but it is thought to result from a complex interaction of environmental and genetic factors.[24] Most commonly patients present with concerns regarding their menstrual cycle or infertility and signs of hyperandrogenism.[24] Because of its variable presentation, diagnosis is a challenge.

The Rotterdam criteria for diagnosis requires two of the three following[24,25]:

   1) Clinical/biochemical hyperandrogenism (hirsutism, increase in terminal hair, acne, central adiposity, alopecia, elevated testosterone)
   2) Ovulatory dysfunction (anovulation or oligomenorrhea)
   3) Polycystic ovaries

Metabolic effects include insulin resistance, impaired glucose tolerance, diabetes, dyslipidemia, and nonalcoholic fatty liver disease (NAFLD), all of which increase the risk of CVD and/or cerebrovascular disease.[25]

The Relationship Between Polycystic Ovary Syndrome and Diabetes

PCOS was originally thought of purely as a reproductive abnormality. Now PCOS is recognized as a nonmodifiable risk factor for diabetes.[24] Patients with PCOS have four times the risk of developing diabetes regardless of BMI and should be screened for diabetes approximately every 1 to 2 years.[22,25]

Insulin resistance is found in 60% to 80% of all patients with PCOS and in 95% of patients with PCOS who are obese.[22] Obesity has an additive effect on glucose metabolism and insulin dysfunction in patients with PCOS. Insulin resistance is postulated to be involved in the development of PCOS by suppressing synthesis of sex hormone–binding globulin and increasing adrenal and ovarian synthesis of androgens, therefore exacerbating hyperandrogenism.[24] Patients with clear hyperandrogenemia have more severe insulin resistance than patients who do not have hyperandrogenemia.[25] Studies suggest an insulin signaling defect in patients with PCOS affects insulin-mediated glucose uptake in adipose and skeletal muscle cells.[25] Decreased secretory response of insulin to meals and higher basal insulin secretion rates are also involved.[22]

As a result, pregnant patients with PCOS have a higher risk of complications and adverse pregnancy outcomes, so it is important for providers to counsel them about these risks.[26]

Combined Treatment of Polycystic Ovary Syndrome and Diabetes

Treatment of PCOS must be individualized.[24] Lifestyle modifications are first-line treatment recommendations for patients with PCOS because diet and exercise improve insulin resistance in patients with PCOS.[22]

For patients who have significant dermatologic or hyperandrogenic symptoms, these are managed with combined oral contraceptive pills and adding an antiandrogen agent, such as spironolactone, for treatment of hirsutism as long as the patient does not desire pregnancy.[26]

Irregular menses and amenorrhea are often associated with decreased fertility, but management depends on desire for pregnancy. For patients who desire pregnancy, clomiphene (an estrogen receptor modulator) or letrozole (an aromatase inhibitor) are recommended.[24,26,27] Metformin has also been used to assist with fertility and menstrual irregularities, but it is less effective and therefore second-line treatment.[24] For patients who do not desire pregnancy, combined oral contraceptive pills are the mainstay of treatment of irregular menses.[24] Little data exist on the long-term risks and benefits of other forms of hormonal contraception.[26]

Metformin should certainly be used in patients with PCOS with insulin resistance because it improves insulin resistance and may reverse impaired glucose tolerance.[22,27] For patients with diabetes with PCOS, metformin is still first-line and other antidiabetic medications are added based on a patient's individual needs and goals. It is important to consider whether a patient desires pregnancy because many diabetes medications are teratogenic.[22]

DYSLIPIDEMIA
Prevalence

Rates of dyslipidemia in the United States have not been rising as steeply as rates of obesity and diabetes, because of greater awareness and effective treatment.[28–30] Global studies listed high low-density lipoproteins (LDL) as the fifth-leading risk factor for all-cause mortality, unchanged from 1990.[30] Regardless of specific lipid levels, around 37% of adults in the United States in recent years have been eligible for cholesterol-lowering medications.[31] Patients with diabetes have a higher prevalence of dyslipidemia.[11]

Overview of the Disease

Dyslipidemias encompass abnormalities of lipoprotein metabolism including elevated levels of total cholesterol (TC), LDL cholesterol, and/or triglycerides and deficient levels of high-density lipoproteins cholesterol. Recommendations for cholesterol-lowering therapy are generally based on total calculated risk of atherosclerotic CVD (ASCVD) adverse events rather than on specific lipid levels.[32] An ASCVD risk calculator is used for this calculation, which includes known history of hypertension and/or diabetes.[11]

Screening for lipid disorders is recommended in all men older than 35 years and in men 20 to 35 years old who have an increased risk for coronary artery disease (CAD).[33] For women, recommendations are to screen in those with increased risk who are older than 20 years.[33]

The Relationship Between Dyslipidemia and Diabetes

Dyslipidemia and diabetes are independent risk factors for ASCVD. Diabetes also has direct effects on dyslipidemia. Patients with diabetes have increased secretion of very low density lipoproteins and abnormal cholesterol transfer leading to changes of LDL particles to small dense LDL, which are more proatherogenic and cause oxidative stress.[31] It has also been found that high-density lipoprotein particles do not prevent oxidation of LDL in patients with diabetes and in those without diabetes.[34]

Poor control of diabetes can persistently worsen dyslipidemic processes because impaired glucose tolerance promotes the formation of atherosclerosis.[35] Diabetes-associated dyslipidemia causes vascular inflammation and other adverse changes that cause progression of atherosclerosis.[36] Patients with diabetes have two to four times the risk of CAD, which is the most serious cause of morbidity and mortality in patients with diabetes.[34]

Combined Treatment of Dyslipidemia and Diabetes

Lipid-lowering therapy decreases the incidence of ASCVD in patients with dyslipidemia but absolute benefits depend on an individual's underlying risk. Patients with higher baseline ASCVD risk, such as patients with diabetes, are more likely to have greater risk reduction.[11,34]

Lifestyle modification through an increase in physical activity and implementing a Mediterranean-style diet or the DASH diet treat dyslipidemia and diabetes.[11] Statin medications reduce ASCVD morbidity and mortality by directly lowering lipid levels and having certain anti-inflammatory and plaque-stabilizing effects.[37]

Statin therapy is recommended by the ADA in addition to lifestyle therapy because it is more effective than lifestyle changes alone.[33] For primary prevention all patients with diabetes aged 40 to 75 without diagnosed ASCVD should use at minimum a moderate-intensity statin medication, whereas for adult patients younger than 40 years statins are added based on individual ASCVD risk. For patients with diabetes with higher ASCVD risk scores, especially risk greater than or equal to 20%, escalation to high-intensity statins is recommended.[11]

For secondary prevention in those with known ASCVD, high-intensity statin therapy is recommended. If patients cannot tolerate the needed statin intensity, the maximally tolerated dose should be used. In patients with diabetes with ASCVD and LDL greater than 70 mg/dL despite maximally tolerated statin, consider additional therapies, such as ezetimibe or PCSK9 inhibitor.[11]

OBSTRUCTIVE SLEEP APNEA
Prevalence

It is estimated between 2% and 14% of the population in the United States has obstructive sleep apnea (OSA) and rates are increasing.[38] Age-adjusted rates of OSA are 4 to 10 times higher with obesity, particularly central obesity.[39]

The prevalence of OSA in patients with diabetes is estimated at 23% but when considering the possibility of undiagnosed individuals the estimated prevalence increases to around 50%.[39]

Overview of the Disease

OSA is a chronic sleep disorder characterized by intermittent hypoxemia and sleep fragmentation caused by recurrent complete or partial obstruction of the upper airway. Predictive clinical features and risk factors include[38]:

- Excessive daytime sleepiness

- Reported gasping during sleep or loud snoring
- Morning headache
- Neck circumference greater than 16 inches
- Family history
- Male sex
- Age older than 50 years
- Commercial motor vehicle driver
- BMI greater than 35
- Postmenopausal women not on hormonal therapy
- Retrognathia
- Preoperative status for bariatric surgery

The validated questionnaire STOP-Bang is a helpful screening tool for OSA that providers can use for patients with suspicious symptoms, especially patients with diabetes given their higher prevalence of OSA.[38,40] Diagnosis requires elevated apnea-hypopnea index calculated in a sleep study.[38] Untreated OSA can lead to many adverse outcomes include hypertension, CVD, diabetes, decreased workplace productivity, and attributable traffic accidents.[40]

The Relationship Between Obstructive Sleep Apnea and Diabetes

OSA is an independent risk factor for diabetes,[40] and they have a bidirectional relationship through chronic inflammation and insulin resistance.[41,42] Studies show patients with OSA have a 37% higher risk of diabetes than patients without OSA when controlling for multiple confounders, and vice versa.[40,42] In patients with diabetes OSA can lead to poor diabetes control, worsened hypertension, CAD, and other microvascular complications.[40]

Studies suggest that recurrent episodes of hypoxemia stimulate the sympathetic system and hypothalamic-adrenal axis, causing increased catecholamine production that then impairs glucose metabolism, reduces insulin sensitivity, and leads to pancreatic β-cell dysfunction.[40,42] Conversely, there are several proposed mechanisms by which diabetes can cause OSA.[40] Diabetic neuropathy is thought specifically to contribute by compromising the autonomic nervous reflexes that protect the upper airway from collapse during sleep.[42]

Combined Treatment of Obstructive Sleep Apnea and Diabetes

Because of the association between sleep apnea and obesity, weight loss and lifestyle changes are recommended. However, although weight loss has been shown to decrease upper airway obstruction, there is less evidence of improvement in general breathing patterns and sleep.[38] Continuous positive airway pressure (CPAP) is the first-line therapy for OSA.[38] CPAP has superior effects on complications of sleep apnea compared with other oral appliances for OSA. CPAP improves sleep indices, reducing blood pressure, increasing left ventricular ejection fraction, and reducing rates of arrhythmia, cardiovascular events, and stroke.[38] Studies have not, however, identified a clear impact of CPAP on glycemic control in diabetes.[43]

NONALCOHOLIC FATTY LIVER DISEASE
Prevalence

It is estimated that globally 25% of adults have NAFLD and the prevalence is increasing.[44,45] In the United States, approximately 30% of all adults have NAFLD.[46] Epidemiologic studies suggest that up to two-thirds of adult patients with diabetes have NAFLD.[45]

Overview of the Disease

NAFLD is defined as excessive deposition of fat in the liver (steatosis) in the absence of other secondary causes. To diagnose NAFLD evidence is needed of hepatic steatosis on liver imaging or liver biopsy histology.

NAFLD is categorized into[44,45]:

- Nonalcoholic fatty liver: $\geq$5% steatosis on histology without signs of hepatocellular injury
- Nonalcoholic steatohepatitis (NASH): $\geq$5% steatosis with signs of hepatocellular injury and inflammation

NASH is a more advanced form of NAFLD associated with fibrosis that carries increased risk of liver cirrhosis and hepatocellular carcinoma.[44]

The pathogenesis of NAFLD is not entirely understood, but involves several metabolic, genetic, environmental, and microbiome mechanisms.[47] Obesity is the most common known risk factor for NAFLD.[45] Adipose cells generate multiple biochemical signals that cause altered metabolism of lipids and glucose that leads to proinflammatory fat accumulation in the liver.[47]

NAFLD is also linked to insulin resistance, central adiposity, hypertension, and dyslipidemia.[48] NAFLD is an independent risk factor for diabetes and CVD. The overall leading cause of death in NAFLD is CVD.[44] Despite all these complications there is not enough evidence for screening recommendations.[46] Providers must therefore remain vigilant and have a high index of suspicion for NAFLD in appropriate patients.[45]

The Relationship Between Nonalcoholic Fatty Liver Disease and Diabetes

Research suggests a bidirectional relationship between NAFLD and diabetes. Because of the lack of screening recommendations, many patients with diabetes are diagnosed with NAFLD long after their diabetes diagnosis, which makes it difficult to study the pathways by which one disease may cause the other.[49] It is proven that insulin resistance has a role in the pathogenesis of NAFLD but the specific mechanisms are unclear.[49]

What is known is that patients with diabetes not only have a higher prevalence of NAFLD, but are more likely to have NASH and advanced fibrosis.[45] Patients with diabetes with NAFLD also have almost twice the risk of ASCVD adverse events than patients with diabetes without NAFLD.[49]

Combined Treatment of Nonalcoholic Fatty Liver Disease and Diabetes

Treatment goals are generally to prevent or reverse hepatic injury and fibrosis. Linked comorbidities (diabetes, hypertension, dyslipidemia, obesity) must also be properly addressed and treated. Weight loss, healthy diet, and adequate exercise are first-line therapies for NAFLD and can also reduce cardiovascular risk.[45,48,50] A meta-analysis found that weight loss of 5% to 10% improved liver histology and normalized liver enzymes in those with abnormal laboratory studies[48]; increased physical activity had a similar effect independent of weight loss.[45,48] Consistent data that diabetes control is more difficult in patients with NAFLD[49] show that the main focus in treating both diseases together is adequate glycemic control and weight loss.

Several systematic reviews did not find sufficient evidence for use of such proposed medications as bile acids and metformin in patients with NAFLD without diabetes.[45,48] However, metformin should be used for treatment of diabetes in NAFLD.[49] Statins are recommended for treatment of concomitant dyslipidemia except if there is decompensated cirrhosis.[45] Thiazolidinediones, such as pioglitazone, improve liver histology in patients with NASH with and without diabetes.[45,50] Benefit of GLP-1s in reducing progression of fibrosis has been found but there is not enough evidence to recommend routine use.[50] Given the currently limited evidence for use of most diabetic medications specifically for NAFLD, larger studies are needed to evaluate utility.[49]

CLINICS CARE POINTS: DIABETIC COMORBIDITIES

- Diabetes-associated conditions (hypertension, obesity, polycystic ovary syndrome, obstructive sleep apnea, dyslipidemia, nonalcoholic fatty liver disease) share pathogenic pathways with diabetes that leads to bidirectional influence.

- All of these conditions recommend lifestyle interventions including appropriate weight loss, diet modifications, and increased physical activity.

- Hypertension is the most common comorbidity with diabetes. First-line medication treatments include angiotensin-converting enzyme inhibitors, angiotensin receptor blockers, calcium channel blockers, and thiazide-type diuretics.

- Obesity is classified according to BMI, and goal of treatment is weight loss.

- Polycystic ovary syndrome is an ovulatory endocrinologic disorder associated with insulin resistance. Treatment can include combined oral contraceptives, spironolactone, metformin, and ovulation inductors.

- Dyslipidemia management is essential to decrease cardiovascular risk. Statin therapy is recommended based on atherosclerotic cardiovascular disease risk.

- Obstructive sleep apnea can lead to multiple cardiovascular adverse events. First-line treatment is continuous positive airway pressure therapy.

- Nonalcoholic fatty liver disease is more likely to be advanced in patients with diabetes. Treatment focuses on lifestyle modification and controlling comorbidities. New possible therapies are being studied.

CONFLICT OF INTEREST

The author has no commercial or financial conflicts of interest.

REFERENCES

1. American Diabetes Association. 8. Obesity management for the treatment of type 2 diabetes: Standards of Medical Care in Diabetes-2021. Diabetes Care 2021; 44(Suppl 1):S100–10.
2. Hypertension. World Health Organization. 2021. Available at: https://www.who.int/news-room/fact-sheets/detail/hypertension.
3. Facts About Hypertension. Centers for Disease Control and Prevention. 2021. Available at: https://www.cdc.gov/bloodpressure/facts.htm. May 22, 2021.
4. Hypertension Prevalence in the U.S.: Million Hearts. Centers for Disease Control and Prevention. 2021. Available at: https://millionhearts.hhs.gov/data-reports/hypertension-prevalence.html. May 22, 2021.
5. Ferrannini E, Cushman WC. Diabetes and hypertension: the bad companions. Lancet 2012;380(9841):601–10.
6. Tsimihodimos V, Gonzalez-Villalpando C, Meigs JB, et al. Hypertension and diabetes mellitus: coprediction and time trajectories. Hypertension 2018;71(3):422–8.
7. American Diabetes Association. 10. Cardiovascular disease and risk management: Standards of Medical Care in Diabetes-2021 [published correction appears in Diabetes Care. 2021 Jun 16]. Diabetes Care 2021;44(Suppl 1):S125–50.

8. James PA, Oparil S, Carter BL, et al. 2014 evidence-based guideline for the management of high blood pressure in adults: report from the panel members appointed to the Eighth Joint National Committee (JNC 8) [published correction appears in JAMA. JAMA 2014;311(5):507–20.

9. Thomopoulos C, Parati G, Zanchetti A. Effects of blood-pressure-lowering treatment on outcome incidence in hypertension: 10 - Should blood pressure management differ in hypertensive patients with and without diabetes mellitus? Overview and meta-analyses of randomized trials. J Hypertens 2017;35(5): 922–44.

10. Unger T, Borghi C, Charchar F, et al. International Society of Hypertension Global Hypertension practice guidelines. J Hypertens 2020;38(6):982–1004.

11. Hypertension: new Guidelines from the International Society of Hypertension. Am Fam Physician 2021;103(12):763–5. Available at: https://www.aafp.org/afp/2021/0615/p763.html. July 18, 2021.

12. Whelton PK, Carey RM, Aronow WS, et al. 2017 ACC/AHA/AAPA/ABC/ACPM/AGS/APhA/ASH/ASPC/NMA/PCNA guideline for the prevention, detection, evaluation, and management of high blood pressure in adults: a report of the American College of Cardiology/American Heart Association Task Force on Clinical Practice Guidelines [published correction appears in J Am Coll Cardiol. 2018 May 15;71(19):2275-2279]. J Am Coll Cardiol 2018;71(19):e127–248.

13. Cryer MJ, Horani T, DiPette DJ. Diabetes and hypertension: a comparative review of current guidelines. J Clin Hypertens (Greenwich) 2016;18(2):95–100.

14. Lastra G, Syed S, Kurukulasuriya LR, et al. Type 2 diabetes mellitus and hypertension: an update. Endocrinol Metab Clin North Am 2014;43(1):103–22.

15. Nutrition, Physical Activity, and Obesity: Data, Trends and Maps. Centers for Disease Control and Prevention. 2021. Available at: https://www.cdc.gov/nccdphp/dnpao/data-trends-maps/index.html. July 12, 2021.

16. Adult Obesity Facts. Centers for Disease Control and Prevention. 2021. Available at: https://www.cdc.gov/obesity/data/adult.html. July 11, 2021.

17. Childhood Obesity Facts. Centers for Disease Control and Prevention. 2021. Available at: https://www.cdc.gov/obesity/data/childhood.html. July 12, 2021.

18. Adult Overweight & Obesity. Centers for Disease Control and Prevention. 2021. Available at: https://www.cdc.gov/obesity/adult/index.html. July 11, 2021.

19. Boles A, Kandimalla R, Reddy PH. Dynamics of diabetes and obesity: epidemiological perspective. Biochim Biophys Acta Mol Basis Dis 2017;1863(5): 1026–36.

20. Greco AV, Mingrone G, Giancaterini A, et al. Insulin resistance in morbid obesity: reversal with intramyocellular fat depletion. Diabetes 2002;51(1):144–51.

21. Choi CHJ, Cohen P. How does obesity lead to insulin resistance? Elife 2017;6: e33298.

22. Lazaridou S, Dinas K, Tziomalos K. Prevalence, pathogenesis and management of prediabetes and type 2 diabetes mellitus in patients with polycystic ovary syndrome. Hormones (Athens) 2017;16(4):373–80.

23. PCOS (Polycystic Ovary Syndrome) and Diabetes. Centers for Disease Control and Prevention. 2020. Available at: https://www.cdc.gov/diabetes/basics/pcos.html. May 28, 2021.

24. Williams T, Mortada R, Porter S. Diagnosis and treatment of polycystic ovary syndrome. Am Fam Physician 2016;94(2):106–13.

25. Rodgers RJ, Avery JC, Moore VM, et al. Complex diseases and co-morbidities: polycystic ovary syndrome and type 2 diabetes mellitus. Endocr Connect 2019;8(3):R71–5.

26. Fauser BC, Tarlatzis BC, Rebar RW, et al. Consensus on women's health aspects of polycystic ovary syndrome (PCOS): the Amsterdam ESHRE/ASRM-Sponsored 3rd PCOS Consensus Workshop Group. Fertil Steril 2012;97(1):28–38.e25.

27. Radosh L. Drug treatments for polycystic ovary syndrome. Am Fam Physician 2009;79(8):671–6.

28. Julson H. Effectiveness of insulin sensitizing drugs for polycystic ovary syndrome. Am Fam Physician 2007;76(9):1308–9.

29. FastStats - Cholesterol. Centers for Disease Control and Prevention. 2021. Available at: https://www.cdc.gov/nchs/fastats/cholesterol.htm. April 29, 2021.

30. Virani SS, Alonso A, Benjamin EJ, et al. Heart disease and stroke statistics—2020 update: a report from the American Heart Association external icon. Circulation 2020;141(9):e139–596.

31. Mercado C, DeSimone AK, Odom E, et al. Prevalence of cholesterol treatment eligibility and medication use among adults—United States, 2005–2012. Morbidity and Mortality Weekly Report 2015;64(47):1305–11. Available at: https://www.cdc.gov/mmwr/preview/mmwrhtml/mm6447a1.htm. April 29, 2021.

32. Last AR, Ference JD, Menzel ER. Hyperlipidemia: drugs for cardiovascular risk reduction in adults. Am Fam Physician 2017;95(2):78–87.

33. Screening for Lipid Disorders in Adults: Recommendation Statement. American Family Physician. 2009. Available at: https://www.aafp.org/afp/2009/1201/p1273.html. May 17, 2021.

34. Beckman JA, Creager MA, Libby P. Diabetes and atherosclerosis: epidemiology, pathophysiology, and management. JAMA 2002;287(19):2570–81.

35. Barzilay JI, Spiekerman CF, Kuller LH, et al. Prevalence of clinical and isolated subclinical cardiovascular disease in older adults with glucose disorders: the Cardiovascular Health Study. Diabetes Care 2001;24(7):1233–9.

36. Fan D, Li L, Li Z, et al. Effect of hyperlipidemia on the incidence of cardio-cerebrovascular events in patients with type 2 diabetes. Lipids Health Dis 2018;17(1):102.

37. Chou R, Dana T, Blazina I, et al. Statins for prevention of cardiovascular disease in adults: evidence report and systematic review for the US Preventive Services Task Force. JAMA 2016;316(19):2008–24.

38. Semelka M, Wilson J, Floyd R. Diagnosis and treatment of obstructive sleep apnea in adults. Am Fam Physician 2016;94(5):355–60.

39. American Diabetes Association. 4. Comprehensive medical evaluation and assessment of comorbidities: Standards of Medical Care in Diabetes-2021. Diabetes Care 2021;44(Suppl 1):S40–52.

40. Subramanian A, Adderley NJ, Tracy A, et al. Risk of incident obstructive sleep apnea among patients with type 2 diabetes. Diabetes Care 2019;42(5):954–63.

41. Foster GD, Sanders MH, Millman R, et al. Obstructive sleep apnea among obese patients with type 2 diabetes. Diabetes Care 2009;32(6):1017–9.

42. Huang T, Lin BM, Stampfer MJ, et al. A population-based study of the bidirectional association between obstructive sleep apnea and type 2 diabetes in three prospective U.S. cohorts. Diabetes Care 2018;41(10):2111–9.

43. Kent BD, McNicholas WT, Ryan S. Insulin resistance, glucose intolerance and diabetes mellitus in obstructive sleep apnoea. J Thorac Dis 2015;7(8):1343–57.

44. Stefan N, Häring HU, Cusi K. Non-alcoholic fatty liver disease: causes, diagnosis, cardiometabolic consequences, and treatment strategies. Lancet Diabetes Endocrinol 2019;7(4):313–24.

45. Chalasani N, Younossi Z, Lavine JE, et al. The diagnosis and management of nonalcoholic fatty liver disease: practice guidance from the American Association for the Study of Liver Diseases. Hepatology 2018;67(1):328–57.

46. Oh RC, Hustead TR. Causes and evaluation of mildly elevated liver transaminase levels. Am Fam Physician 2011;84(9):1003–8.

47. Rinella ME. Nonalcoholic fatty liver disease: a systematic review [published correction appears in JAMA. 2015]. JAMA 2015;313(22):2263–73.

48. Wilkins T, Tadkod A, Hepburn I, et al. Nonalcoholic fatty liver disease: diagnosis and management. Am Fam Physician 2013;88(1):35–42.

49. Hazlehurst JM, Woods C, Marjot T, et al. Non-alcoholic fatty liver disease and diabetes. Metabolism 2016;65(8):1096–108.

50. Leoni S, Tovoli F, Napoli L, et al. Current guidelines for the management of non-alcoholic fatty liver disease: a systematic review with comparative analysis. World J Gastroenterol 2018;24(30):3361–73.

Diabetes in Pregnancy: Preconception to Postpartum

Amber M. Healy, DO

KEYWORDS

- Pre-gestational diabetes • Gestational diabetes • Pregnancy • Preconception

KEY POINTS

- Diabetes control is an important part of preconception counseling in women with diabetes to prevent adverse outcomes.
- Insulin is the preferred treatment in pregestational and gestational diabetes
- Screening for gestational diabetes is still recommended between 24 and 28 weeks gestation in one of the 2 different ways.
- Insulin doses require adjustment and close follow-up in pregnancy to maintain adequate control as insulin sensitivity changes throughout pregnancy.
- Women with gestational diabetes require continuous, routine screening after delivery as the risk of developing diabetes increases with time.

INTRODUCTION

Diabetes in pregnancy, which can be further defined as pregestational diabetes in pregnancy or gestational diabetes mellitus (GDM), is estimated to affect up to 10% of pregnancies in the United States (US).[1] Pregestational diabetes can be either type 1 diabetes, type 2 diabetes, diabetes from underlying genetic causes, diabetes from exocrine pancreatic disorders (eg, pancreatitis), or drug/chemical induced diabetes as seen with organ transplants and antiretroviral therapy for HIV that a woman has before becoming pregnant.[2] Gestational diabetes is diabetes that is diagnosed in pregnancy, usually during the second trimester. Undiagnosed diabetes found in the first trimester during initial prenatal laboratories is more likely pregestational diabetes that had not been recognized previously. Roughly 1% to 2% of pregnancies are affected by type 1 or type 2 diabetes and 6% to 9% of pregnant women develop gestational diabetes.[1] Diabetes in pregnancy, whether it is pregestational or gestational, can lead to adverse outcomes for both mother and offspring throughout the pregnancy. Close monitoring and follow-up are important in minimizing adverse outcomes and complications.

Ohio University Heritage College of Osteopathic Medicine (OUHCOM) and Ohio Health O'Bless Hospital, OUHCOM, Heritage Hall 348C, 191 West Union Street, 1 Ohio University, Athens, OH 45701, USA
E-mail address: holdera@ohio.edu

Prim Care Clin Office Pract 49 (2022) 287–300
https://doi.org/10.1016/j.pop.2021.11.009
0095-4543/22/© 2021 Elsevier Inc. All rights reserved.
primarycare.theclinics.com

PREEXISTING DIABETES IN PREGNANCY

Reportedly 45% of pregnancies in the United States are unplanned.[3] Rates of preexisting diabetes have increased, including both type 1 and type 2.[4] To decrease the risk of adverse pregnancy outcomes, women with diabetes considering pregnancy require tighter glucose control and medication review before trying to conceive. The American Diabetes Association (ADA) Standards of Care recommend that preconception counseling start at puberty and continue for all women of child-bearing age.[5] Family planning discussions should occur and contraception should be prescribed until diabetes control is optimized for pregnancy.[5] Preconception counseling should be tailored to the type of diabetes as women with type 1 diabetes are treated with insulin and women with type 2 diabetes are treated with different combinations of lifestyle, insulin, oral hypoglycemics, and noninsulin injectable medications. Medications used for both diabetes and its comorbid conditions require review and adjustment in pregnancy, based on their safety profiles. Some medications need to be stopped or changed to safer alternatives. Poor blood sugar control can lead to adverse maternal and neonatal outcomes, which also needs to be addressed as part of a preconception checklist. See **Table 1**.[5–7]

The effects of hyperglycemia on a fetus can lead to congenital abnormalities, spontaneous abortion, preterm delivery, and macrosomia. Congenital abnormalities can occur in multiple organ systems. See **Table 2**.[8] Most of the congenital malformations have been shown to occur before the seventh week of gestation,[9] which is within the time frame for organogenesis. A hemoglobin A1c (HbA1c) goal of 6.0% to 6.5% before conception is ideal unless maternal hypoglycemia is of concern. In that case, the HbA1c target can be individualized to 7% or less.[5] Maternal consequences of hyperglycemia in pregnancy can include:

Table 1 Preconception checklist	
Medical History	☐ Review Current Medications[a] ☐ Review Family and Genetic History ☐ Immunizations ☐ Obstetric and Gynecologic History ☐ HIV status ☐ Infectious Disease Screening
Self-Care/Social History	☐ Substance Abuse History ☐ Domestic Violence Abuse History ☐ Maintenance and achievement of body weight[b] ☐ Nutrition [c] ☐ Exercise[d] ☐ Teratogen Exposure
Pregestational Diabetes Specific	☐ Hemoglobin A1c goal <6.0%–6.5% ☐ Thyroid function (TSH <2.5 mIU/L) ☐ Retinal examination ☐ 24 h urine for protein ☐ EKG (over age 35)

[a] Medications that are teratogenic need to be stopped (ACE inhibitors, ARBs, statins).
[b] Weight management is important in pregestational diabetes but is also important in obese women who are at higher risk of developing gestational diabetes.
[c] Vitamins are important especially folic acid. A prenatal vitamin with 400mcg of folic acid is recommended. Vitamins: B12, A, C, and D as well as calcium should also be a part of the vitamin. Limiting caffeine is also important.
[d] 150 mins of weekly exercise which is 30 min 5 d per week

Table 2
Congenital abnormalities that can occur due to hyperglycemia in women with pregestational diabetes

Body System	Specific Conditions
Central Nervous System	anencephaly spina bifida microcephaly neural tube defect holoprosencephaly caudal regression syndrome
Musculoskeletal	sacral agenesis limb defects atrial septal defects coarctation of the aorta
Cardiovascular	transposition of great vessels ventricular septal defects cardiomyopathy single umbilical artery renal agenesis
Urogenital	hydronephrosis ureteric abnormalities duodenal atresia
Gastrointestinal	anorectal atresia small left colon syndrome

- Miscarriage
- Preeclampsia/eclampsia
- Diabetic ketoacidosis (DKA)
- Worsening of underlying retinopathy, nephropathy, and neuropathy
- Cesarean section (C-section)

Possible adverse neonatal outcomes:

- Short-term
  - Macrosomia → birth injury (eg, shoulder dystocia, clavicular fracture), cesarean section
  - Intrauterine Growth Restriction
  - Neonatal hypoglycemia
  - Stillbirth
  - Preterm delivery
  - Respiratory distress
- Long-term
  - Childhood obesity[10]
  - Impaired glucose tolerance[10]
  - Development of cardiovascular disease[10]
  - Female offspring more likely to have GDM in their own pregnancies[10]

Type 1 Diabetes Mellitus and Pregnancy

In the United States, pregnancies complicated by type 1 diabetes mellitus continue to increase; in 2010 the estimate was 0.2% to 0.5% of all pregnancies.[11] Type 1 diabetes is a condition of the pancreatic beta cells not producing insulin, either from autoimmune destruction or direct viral destruction of the beta cells. This process tends to occur earlier in life, affecting women of childbearing age. Women with type 1 diabetes are already on insulin before pregnancy. Ensuring that the insulin regimen is reviewed and is safe before conception is important. See **Table 3**.[12–26] Women with type 1 diabetes before pregnancy need counseling as outlined previously to ensure the best chance of positive outcomes for the mother and infant. The preconception HbA1c goal is 6.5% or less. During the second and third trimesters of pregnancy, the HbA1c goal is 6.0% or less, if achievable without hypoglycemia.[5] Women can be managed with either multiple daily injections (MDI) or by continuous subcutaneous infusion of insulin (CSII) via an insulin pump. One head-to-head trial indicated that women treated with MDI tend to have less maternal hyperglycemia, less NICU time, and less neonatal hypoglycemia compared with CSII.[27] However, the differences between MDI and CSII groups with respect to C-section rates, birth weight, and birth injury were not statistically significant.[27]

Glucose and insulin requirements change throughout pregnancy. In the first-trimester insulin resistance improves and women may find that they require less insulin to maintain glycemic control.[28] During the second and third-trimester insulin resistance increases due to increased production of placental hormones and insulin requirements increase to maintain blood glucose targets.[29] This can lead to patients requiring a 9% to 36% increase in insulin.[30] (**Table 4**: Blood glucose targets in pregnancy,[5] **Table 5**: CGMs target ranges in pregnancy[31]) After delivery, insulin resistance decreases. As a result, insulin doses should be decreased by 20% to 40% with further

Table 3 Insulin safety in pregnancy		
Insulin Type	**Safety in Pregnancy**	**Lactation Safety**
insulin aspart niacinamide	Not studied in humans	Not studied
insulin lispro aabc	Not studied in humans	Not studied
inhaled regular insulin	Category C[c]	excreted in milk in breast milk in animal studies
insulin aspart[a]	Category B[b]	excreted in breast milk[d]
insulin glulisine[a]	Category C[c]	excreted in breast milk[d]
insulin lispro[a] (U-100/U-200)	Category B[b]	excreted in breast milk[d]
insulin regular U-100[a]	Category B[b]	excreted in breast milk[d]
insulin regular U-500[a]	Category B[b]	excreted in breast milk[d]
NPH insulin[a]	Category B[b]	excreted in breast milk[d]
degludec[a] (U100/U-200)	Category C[c]	excreted in breast milk in animal studies
detemir[a]	Category B[c]	excreted in breast milk[d]
glargine[a] (U-100)	Category C[c]	
glargine (U-300)	No human studies	excretion in breast milk unknown

Of note, categories were removed and now the FDA requires a summary of risks in pregnancy and lactation (12). Categories are here for historic reference regarding safety.
  [a] Human Studies to date do not indicate insulin causes adverse maternal or fetal outcomes
  [b] Category B previous classification used by FDA: Controlled studies in animals or pregnant have not shown risk to the fetus. (FDA) Generally considered safe.
  [c] Category C previous classification used by FDA: controlled animal studies showed adverse effects to fetus, no studies in women. (FDA) Used when maternal benefit outweighs risk to fetus.
  [d] Risk to infant not studied benefit to breastfeeding and mother's clinical needs should be considered.

Table 4
Glucose targets in pregnancy

	Glucose Target
Fasting blood sugar	<95 mg/dL
1-h postprandial	110–140 mg/dL
2-h postprandial	100–120 mg/dL

(*Data from* 14. Management of Diabetes in Pregnancy: Standards of Medical Care in Diabetes—2021. Diabetes Care.2021:44(S1))

reduction as needed for maternal hypoglycemia.[32] Lactation can cause further hypoglycemia necessitating further insulin adjustments.

Type 2 Diabetes Mellitus and Pregnancy

The number of people diagnosed with type 2 diabetes continues to increase while the age of diagnosis has been decreasing.[33] As a result, more women of child-bearing age have type 2 diabetes diagnosed before conception or early in pregnancy. One study showed a 367% increase in deliveries affected by type 2 diabetes between 1994 and 2004.[34] Type 2 diabetes is a result of beta cells ineffectively secreting insulin and decreased sensitivity in insulin-sensitive tissues (ie, insulin resistance) leading to hyperglycemia.[35] Treatment options for type 2 diabetes include pills, insulins, and glucagon-like peptide-1 receptor agonists (GLP-1RA). Not all of these choices are safe in pregnancy and most have not been studied in pregnancy, making insulin the preferred treatment of type 2 diabetes in pregnancy just as insulin is preferred with type 1 diabetes. Historically, metformin and glyburide have been used as treatments for type 2 diabetes in pregnancy. While metformin continues to be used, glyburide is no longer used as frequently. A meta-analysis demonstrated an increased risk of fetal macrosomia and neonatal hypoglycemia compared with insulin and favored metformin for an oral agent.[36] Other studies have demonstrated benefits to metformin use in pregnancy. Feig and colleagues[37] showed that neonatal composite outcomes were not different in women who received metformin versus those who did not receive metformin in addition to insulin for T2DM in pregnancy. However, women who received metformin had better glucose control, gained less weight, required less insulin, and had fewer C-sections.[37] Another study also showed there was no difference in the neonatal composite outcomes and less maternal weight gain in women treated with metformin versus insulin.[38] This same group followed offspring to the age of 2 and collected data regarding body composition, finding no difference in BMI, total body fat, percentage body fat, central-to-peripheral fat, or DEXA-calculated abdominal-thigh-fat ratios between the

Table 5
Glucose targets on CGMs

	Time Goal	Glucose Range
Time above Range	<25%	>140 mg/dL
Time in Range	70% or more	63–140 mg/dL
Time below Range	<4%	<63 mg/dL
	<1%	<54 mg/dL

(*Data from* Battelino T, Danne T, Bergenstal RM, et al. Clinical targets for continuous glucose monitoring data interpretation: recommendations from the international consensus on time in range. Diabetes Care 2019;42:1593–1603)

metformin and insulin-treated groups.[39] Children exposed to metformin in utero were found to have larger upper arm circumferences, bigger biceps, and subscapular skinfolds indicating more subcutaneous fat stores.[39] This would indicate a fat distribution that could promote better insulin sensitivity favoring the use of metformin in treating diabetes in pregnancy. Also, when metformin is taken before conception by women with polycystic ovarian syndrome, it has been shown to decrease miscarriage when continued through 12 weeks gestation.[40] For this reason many clinicians will continue metformin through the first trimester in women with type 2 diabetes. However, ACOG recommends limiting the use of oral diabetes agents, with the caveat that they can be considered when individualizing therapy to the patient.[7] The ADA Standards of Care also recommends insulin first-line and oral agents in some cases whereby the patient may have barriers to following an insulin regimen.[5]

Some women with type 2 diabetes may be managed on oral agents before pregnancy, although as mentioned earlier switching to insulin is preferred. While NPH is a more traditional insulin choice, detemir is also an option in pregnancy. Prandial insulin should be 50% of the total daily insulin dose and the other 50% should be given as basal insulin. The recommended insulin dose varies by trimester and is based on actual body weight (kg) as listed later in discussion:

- First trimester: 0.6–0.7 units/kg/day[41–43]
- Second trimester: 0.8 units/kg/day[41–43]
- Third trimester: 0.9 to 1 units/kg/day[41–43]

Women with type 2 diabetes have an increased risk of blood pressure issues in pregnancy. First-line antihypertensive agents used to treat hypertension (eg, angiotensin-converting enzyme inhibitors and angiotensin receptor blockers) are contraindicated in pregnancy due to teratogenicity. Drugs that can be used to treat hypertension in pregnancy include methyldopa, labetalol, and long-acting nifedipine.[44] Blood pressure goals are 110 to 135/85 mmHg in pregnancy.[44]

When women are treated for hyperlipidemia they cannot use statins due to teratogenicity. Ezetimibe, niacin, and fenofibrate also should not be used in pregnancy. If a woman requires continued treatment of hyperlipidemia, bile acid sequestrants can be used to treat low density lipoprotein (LDL) cholesterol and omega-3 fatty acids can be used to treat triglycerides.[45]

Other Considerations in Pregestational Diabetes

Glucose monitoring should occur at least six times per day, including before and after meals and as needed.[41] The goal is to capture fasting, postprandial, and bedtime readings to optimize insulin dosing to reach blood sugar goals (see **Table 4**).[5] Continuous glucose monitoring system (CGMS) use in pregnancy, while endorsed by professional organizations, is not approved by the FDA. However, it can be used to see time in range targets to assess glycemic control (see **Table 5**).[32]

The effects of morning sickness and food aversions on blood sugar control and insulin requirements must be considered in the management of preexisting diabetes in pregnancy. Morning sickness is nausea and/or vomiting that occurs during pregnancy and it is most likely to occur during the first trimester, usually before 9 weeks gestation.[46] Nausea can lead to decreased food intake and can be a symptom of hypoglycemia. Vomiting, when intractable, causes dehydration.[46] Hypoglycemia risks are increased with vomiting when an insulin dose meant to cover consumed carbohydrates is still present while the carbohydrates have been expelled through vomiting. Because of the hypoglycemic risk, patients need to monitor blood sugar more closely. Women with type 1 diabetes who have vomited should also be advised to monitor ketone levels frequently as nausea and vomiting are also symptoms of DKA.[47] Patients with morning sickness should eat 6 small meals per day and avoid fatty foods, spicy foods, and caffeine.[47] Women requiring insulin should take rapid-acting insulin after eating once the blood sugar starts to rise.[47] After vomiting, fluids with carbohydrate content can be substituted in place of food as they may be better tolerated. Then patients can resume eating.

Preeclampsia and Aspirin

Preexisting diabetes, type 1 or 2, is a risk factor for preeclampsia. Aspirin has been shown to reduce this risk. Therefore, it is recommended that women with pregestational diabetes take 60 mg to 162 mg of aspirin daily, initiated between 12 and 16 weeks gestation, as prophylaxis against preeclampsia.[48,49]

GESTATIONAL DIABETES MELLITUS

Gestational diabetes mellitus (GDM) is defined as diabetes that is first diagnosed in pregnancy, usually toward the end of the second trimester. It is estimated that GDM affects up to 10% of pregnancies in the US.[1] The USPSTF recommends that screening for GDM occurs between 24 and 28 weeks gestation.[50] Due to the increasing prevalence of diabetes, there is some debate that screening should occur earlier than 24 weeks gestation to look for undiagnosed pregestational diabetes. However, the best screening option has not been determined and there is no consensus on the diagnostic criteria for these tests. The percentage of women with GDM who have hyperglycemia before 24 weeks has been estimated to be 15% to 70%, so earlier screening for GDM is also under consideration.[51] Options for screening include HbA1c, OGTT, or fasting plasma glucose drawn with initial prenatal laboratories in women with risk factors for GDM. There is not a clear HbA1c diagnostic value for treatment, although most experts suggest 5.9%. One study identified all women with diabetes enrolled with hemoglobin A1c of 5.9% or higher during the first trimester.[52] A fasting plasma glucose level of 110 mg/dL had the highest specificity early in pregnancy, while 92 mg/dL had a high false-positive rate.[50] OGTT, if negative early in pregnancy, still needs to be repeated later in pregnancy (between 24 and 28 weeks). Research has been inconclusive about the benefit of earlier treatment of GDM due to concerns about overtreatment. Nevertheless, many experts agree that women with risk factors for GDM should be screened in the first trimester.

Risk factors for GDM include:[53]

- Age (over 35 years)
- Overweight or obesity
- Excessive weight gain in pregnancy
- Central body fat deposition
- Family history of diabetes
- Short stature (less than five feet)
- Excessive fetal growth
- Polyhydramnios
- Hypertension or preeclampsia in the current pregnancy
- History of recurrent miscarriage
- Offspring malformation
- Fetal or neonatal death
- Macrosomia
- Previous GDM
- Polycystic ovarian syndrome

Diagnosis of GDM is made one of the 2 ways, but neither test is considered the gold standard. There is a one-step oral glucose tolerance test (OGTT) and a two-step OGTT to diagnose GDM. The one-step OGTT is a test whereby the patient does not eat for 8 hours before the test and a fasting glucose reading is drawn, then the patient drinks a 75g dextrose drink and then has her glucose level drawn at 1 hour after drinking the dextrose and again at 2 hours.[5,54] Diagnosis of GDM is made if fasting blood glucose is more than 92 mg/dL, 1-h blood glucose is more than 180 mg/dL, or 2-h blood glucose is more than 153 mg/dL.[5] The two-step OGTT involves an initial 1-hour test whereby the patient is not required to fast. She is given a 50g dextrose drink and has her glucose drawn an hour later.[55] If her results show glucose of less than 140 mg/dL, then she has screened negative for GDM. However, if her results reveal a glucose level greater than 140 mg/dL, then she should complete a 3-hour OGTT test whereby she is given a 100 g dextrose drink and blood glucose levels are checked fasting, 1 hour, 2 hours, and 3 hours after consuming the dextrose. A positive diagnosis is made if 2 of the 4 readings are elevated, which is fasting greater than or equal to 95 mg/dL, 1 hour at least 180 mg/dL, 2 hours at least 155 mg/dL, and 3 hours at least 140 mg/dL. Neither modality of screening has been shown to be more effective at diagnosing gestational diabetes.[56] More women are diagnosed with the one-step method of testing which catches more women with mild hyperglycemia. However, there was not a statistically significant difference between the 2 groups with respect to maternal and fetal outcomes.[56]

Initial treatment of GDM includes diet, physical activity, and self-monitoring of blood glucose (SMBG). Dietary recommendations for GDM include 3 meals and 2 to 4 snacks per day with the timing of intake individualized to the patient including 175 g of carbohydrates per day, 71 g of protein and 28 g of fiber.[57] Physical activity is recommended, but initiating intense activity in pregnancy is not indicated. Walking can be tolerated by most pregnant women and initiating a walking routine can benefit glucose control.[57] SMBG should occur four times daily, fasting and then 1 or 2 hours postprandially. Targets of less than 95 mg/dL fasting, less than 140 mg/dL 1 hour postprandial or less than 120 mg/dL 2 hours postprandial. Of note, the 1 hour or 2 hours postprandial timing starts with the first bite of food of a meal. If blood glucose levels are not at goal, then medication may be needed to treat GDM. Insulin is the preferred treatment in GDM, just as it is with pregestational diabetes. Oral agents can be used in some cases, as aforementioned.

DELIVERY

Recommendations for insulin and other medication use before delivery depend on the type of diabetes. Women with type 1 diabetes cannot stop their insulin due to the risk of DKA. Keeping glucose tightly controlled is important in women with both type 1 and type 2 diabetes to prevent neonatal hypoglycemia with higher maternal blood glucose before delivery. Insulin drips can and should be used during labor and delivery. While on an insulin drip blood sugar needs to be monitored, typically every 2 to 4 hours during the latent phase of labor and every 1 to 2 hours in the active phase of labor.[32] More insulin is required during the latent phase of spontaneous labor with insulin requirements dropping to nearly zero during the active phase of delivery.[32] Keeping the insulin drip titrated to blood sugars of 70 to 140 mg/dL is the goal during delivery, sometimes requiring supplementation with 5% dextrose when the blood sugar drops less than 100 mg/dL.[32] GDM, when well controlled by diet alone, does not require an insulin drip. Women undergoing planned C- section should take their usual night-time dose of insulin and then not use their morning insulin dose if the procedure can be performed early in the morning. However, if the C-section is planned for later in the day, the morning dose of NPH should be administered and corrective dose insulin used as needed.[32] Alternatively, an insulin drip with 5% dextrose can be initiated to prevent ketosis.[32] Women taking insulin detemir would already have their basal insulin on board so rapid-acting correction insulin as needed could be used. A similar approach would be considered in the induction of labor in terms of insulin dosing and adjustment. Women on insulin pumps can be advised to continue current rates overnight and then can continue basal rates in the morning in the anticipation of delivery. If there is a problem with morning hypoglycemia, basal rates can be decreased so that the patient receives less insulin.[58] Correction boluses may be taken as needed before the C-section as with other surgeries lasting less than 2 hours.[58] Oral diabetes agents would be held the morning of the C-section or induction.

After delivery, insulin requirements will change. Women with pregestational diabetes will typically see a reduction in insulin requirements after the placenta is delivered and may not require insulin immediately after delivery. However, women with type 1 diabetes should not omit insulin (to prevent DKA). Options for postpregnancy insulin dosing are: 0.6 units per kg/day, one-third to one-half of the pregnancy dose, or resuming prepregnancy insulin doses if known.[59] Insulin sensitivity returns to prepregnancy levels in one to 2 weeks after delivery. Women with GDM should also see their insulin resistance return to normal after delivery and can discontinue insulin after delivery (if it was required during pregnancy).

POSTPARTUM

Contraception and family planning should be addressed to prevent unplanned pregnancies and help with spacing between pregnancies. Women with diabetes can be offered the same options for contraception as women without diabetes. Women with GDM are 50% more likely to have shorter interpregnancy intervals compared with women without GDM.[60] Interpregnancy intervals of less than 18 months have been associated with worse perinatal outcomes. This makes contraception counseling more important.

Screening and follow-up for type 2 diabetes in women with GDM is recommended to occur via OGTT between 4 and 12 weeks postpartum.[5] A 2-hour OGTT test with a 75g dextrose load is the test of choice. The diagnostic criteria for prediabetes and diabetes are the same as they would be for a nonpregnant woman at this time (**Table 6**).[2] Women with a previous history of GDM should be counseled to have screening completed everyone to 3 years, which can be conducted as a yearly hemoglobin A1c or fasting plasma glucose, or a 75g OGTT completed every 3 years.[5] It is also beneficial to consider referring the patient to the National Diabetes Prevention Program. Women with GDM are eligible to enroll in this program and its lifestyle

Table 6				
Diagnostic criteria in nonpregnant individuals				
		Normal	**Prediabetes**	**Diabetes**
OGTT[a]	fasting	<100 mg/dL	101–125 mg/dL	>126 mg/dL
	2 h	<140 mg/dL	140–199 mg/dL	>200 mg/dL
Laboratory	HbA1c[b]	<5.6%	5.7%-6.4%	>6.5%

Prediabetes is further subcategorized with fasting laboratory values in the prediabetes range indicating impaired fasting glucose and laboratories values at 2 h in the prediabetes range indicating impaired glucose tolerance.
[a] OGTT, oral glucose tolerance test.
[b] HbA1c, hemoglobin A1c.

modifications have shown benefit in reducing diabetes by 35%.[61] Metformin has been shown to reduce progression to type 2 diabetes by 40%.[61] Lifetime risk of progression to diabetes increases with time in a linear pattern with up to 60% increased risk identified at 50 years.[62] A study from Finland demonstrated that up to 7 years after GDM diagnosis 5.7% of women developed type 1 diabetes and, consistent with previous statistics, 60.9% developed type 2 diabetes.[63] In women who have had GDM continued, regular, monitoring continues to be important as it not only increases the chances of developing type 2 diabetes but also hypertension, nonalcoholic fatty liver disease, and cardiovascular disease.[64]

Lactation

Breastfeeding should be encouraged in women with GDM and pregestational diabetes, due to its benefits for both mother and baby. Metabolic benefits, including decreases in lipid and glucose levels, have been seen in women with GDM who breastfeed more than 3 months.[65] Women with pregestational diabetes and GDM can have delayed lactogenesis and be slower to produce more copious amounts of breast milk, so breastfeeding may be challenging early after delivery.[66] To minimize the risk of neonatal hypoglycemia, early and frequent feedings are recommended.[66] In women with pregestational diabetes, lactation can affect glycemic control and insulin dosing may require adjustment.[5] Maternal hypoglycemia tends to occur about an hour after breastfeeding, so counsel patients to consume a snack during breastfeeding to prevent this and to prevent frequent insulin adjustments.[59] The risk of nocturnal hypoglycemia also increases, possibly requiring insulin dose adjustment for prevention.

Women with type 1 diabetes will continue to be managed on insulin; however, women with type 2 diabetes have other options for diabetes treatment. The use of oral hypoglycemics or noninsulin injectable medications is dependent on breastfeeding status. Safety of medications during lactation is variable between classes. Metformin and secretagogues are considered generally safe, while other medication classes lack the research to demonstrate safety with lactation, so should be avoided until the infant is weaned.

SUMMARY

Diabetes can affect pregnancy at conception if preexistent as either type 1 or type 2 diabetes, so tight control should be included as part of preconception counseling. GDM is diagnosed at 24 to 28 weeks gestation via OGTT, but there is debate over whether or not screening should occur earlier than 24 weeks, and there are 2 options for screening. The preferred treatment of preexisting diabetes in pregnancy is insulin. Women with preexisting type 2 diabetes may also take metformin, depending on circumstances, and research has shown benefits to both the mother and baby. Diet is the first-line treatment of GDM, but insulin is preferred when needed. Insulin needs change through pregnancy and after delivery so constant adjustment and frequent follow-up are necessary. After delivery insulin is stopped in GDM while insulin is usually reduced in women with pregestational diabetes. Additional insulin reduction may be needed with lactation. Regular screening for diabetes after pregnancy in women with GDM is necessary as the risk of developing diabetes is increased.

CLINICS CARE POINTS

- Screening for diabetes gestational in the first trimester is an opportunity to diagnose glycemic issues early in women with risk factors. Fasting plasma glucose or hemoglobin A1c would be the easiest to obtain with values of 110 mg/dL or hemoglobin A1c of 5.9% being the most sensitive and specific to diagnose gestational diabetes

- Metformin use should be continued through 12 week gestation if taken at the time of conception and stopped per some experts; however, benefits of metformin taken longer during pregnancy have been seen in both mother and baby, so metformin can be taken longer in pregnancy.
- While the one-step OGTT diagnoses more mild gestational diabetes, neither the one-step nor the two-step OGTTs are better for neonatal outcomes so ordering either test to screen for gestational diabetes is acceptable.

DISCLOSURE

Dr A.M. Healy has no conflicts of interest or financial disclosures that are relevant to this manuscript.

REFERENCES

1. Centers for Disease Control and Prevention. Gestational diabetes. 2020. Available at: https://www.cdc.gov/diabetes/basics/gestational. April 15, 2021.
2. American Diabetes Association. Classification and diagnosis of diabetes: standards of medical care—2021. Diabetes Care 2021;44(S1):S15–33. https://doi.org/10.2337/dc21-S002.
3. Finer LB, Zolna MR. Declines in unintended pregnancy in the United States, 2008-2011. N Engl J Med 2016;374(9):843–52. https://doi.org/10.1056/NEJMsa1506575.
4. Simmons D. Paradigm shifts in the management of diabetes in pregnancy: the importance of type 2 diabetes and early hyperglycemia in pregnancy: the Norbert Freinkel Award lecture. Diabetes Care 2021;44(5):1075–81.
5. 14. Management of diabetes in pregnancy: standards of medical care in diabetes—2021. Diabetes Care 2021;44(S1):S200–10.
6. American College of Gynecology. Prepregnancy counseling. Obstet Gynecol 2019;133(1):12.
7. American College of Gynecology. Practice bulletin 201: prepregnancy diabetes mellitus. Obstet Gynecol 2018;132(6):e228–48.
8. Chen CP. Congenital malformations associated with maternal diabetes. Taiwanese J Obstet Gynecol 2005;44(1):1–7.
9. Mills JL, Baker L, Goldman AS. Malformations in infants of diabetic mothers occur before the seventh gestational week: implications for treatment. Diabetes 1979;28:292–3.
10. Plows JF, Stanley JL, Baker PN, et al. The pathophysiology of gestational diabetes mellitus. Int J Mol Sci 2018;19(3342). https://doi.org/10.3390/ijms19113342.
11. Vargas R, Repke JT, Ural SH. Type 1 diabetes mellitus in pregnancy. Rev Obstet Gynecol 2010;3(3):92–100.
12. Food and Drug Administration. Content and format of labeling for human prescription drug and biological products; requirements for pregnancy and lactation labeling. Final rule. Fed Regist 2014;79(233):72063–103.
13. PI Lyumjev. Available at: http://pi.lilly.com/us/lyumjev-uspi.pdf. March 21, 2021.
14. PI Fiasp. Available at: https://www.novo-pi.com/fiasp.pdf. March 21, 2021.
15. PI Afrezza. Available at: https://www.accessdata.fda.gov/drugsatfda_docs/label/2014/022472lbl.pdf. March 21, 2021.
16. PI Novolog. Available at: https://www.novo-pi.com/insulinaspart.pdf. March 21, 2021.

17. PI Apidra. Available at: https://products.sanofi.us/Apidra/apidra.html#section-10. 3. March 2021.
18. PI Humalog. Available at: https://pi.lilly.com/us/humalog-pen-pi.pdf. March 21, 2021.
19. PI Novolin R. Available at: https://www.novo-pi.com/novolinr.pdf. March 21, 2021.
20. PI Humulin R U-500. Available at: https://pi.lilly.com/us/humulin-r-u500-pi.pdf. March 21, 2021.
21. PI Humulin N. Available at: http://pi.lilly.com/us/HUMULIN-N-USPI.pdf. March 21, 2021.
22. PI Tresiba. Available at: https://www.novo-pi.com/tresiba.pdf. March 21, 2021.
23. PI Levemir. Available at: https://www.novo-pi.com/levemir.pdf. March 21, 2021.
24. PI Basaglar. Available at: http://pi.lilly.com/us/basaglar-uspi.pdf. March 21, 2021.
25. PI Lantus. Available at: https://products.sanofi.us/lantus/lantus.html#section-10. 1. March 21, 2021.
26. PI Toujeo. Available at: https://www.accessdata.fda.gov/drugsatfda_docs/label/2015/206538lbl.pdf. March 21, 2021.
27. Feig DS, Corcoy R, Donovan LE, et al. Pumps or multiple daily injections in pregnancy involving type 1 diabetes: a prespecified analysis of the CONCEPTT randomized trial. Diabetes Care 2018;41:2471–9. https://doi.org/10.2337/dc18-1437.
28. García-Patterson A, Gich I, Amini SB, et al. Insulin requirements throughout pregnancy in women with type 1 diabetes mellitus: three changes of direction. Diabetologia 2010;53:446–51. https://doi.org/10.1007/s00125-009-1633-z.
29. Kampmann U, Knorr S, Fuglsang J, et al. Determinants of maternal insulin resistance during pregnancy: an updated review. J Diabetes Res 2019;2019:5320156.
30. Skajaa GØ, Fuglsang J, Kampmann U, et al. Parity increases insulin requirements in pregnant women with type 1 diabetes. J Clin Endocrinol Metab 2018;103(6): 2302–8.
31. Battelino T, Danne T, Bergenstal RM, et al. Clinical targets for continuous glucose monitoring data interpretation: recommendations from the international consensus on time in range. Diabetes Care 2019;42:1593–603.
32. Kalra P, Anakal M. Peripartum management of diabetes. Indian J Endocrinol Metab 2013;17(Suppl1):S72–6.
33. Mayer-Davis E, Lawrence JM, Dabelea D, et al. Incidence trends of type 1 and type 2 diabetes among youths, 2002-2012. N Eng J Med 2017;376(15):1419–29.
34. Albrecht SS, Kuklina EV, Bansil P, et al. Diabetes trends among delivery hospitalizations in the U.S., 1994-2004. Diabetes Care 2010;33:768–73.
35. Galicia-Garcia U, Benito-Vicente A, Jebari S, et al. Pathophysiology of type 2 diabetes mellitus. Int J Mol Sci 2020;21(17):6275. https://doi.org/10.3390/ijms21176275.
36. Poolsup N, Suksomboon N, Amin M. Efficacy and safety of oral antidiabetic drugs in comparison to insulin in treating gestational diabetes mellitus: a meta-analysis. PLoS One 2014;9(10):e109985. https://doi.org/10.1371/journal.pone.0109985.
37. Feig DS, Donovan LE, Zinman B, et al. Metformin in women with type 2 diabetes on pregnancy (MiTy): a multicenter, international, randomized, placebo-controlled trial. Lancet Diabetes Endocrinol 2020;8(10):834–44. https://doi.org/10.1016/S2213-8587(2)30310-7.
38. Rowan JA, Battin MR. Metformin versus insulin for the treatment of gestational diabetes. N Engl J Med 2008;358:2003–15. https://doi.org/10.1056/MEJMoa0707193.

39. Rowan JA, Rush EC, Obolonkin V, et al. Metformin in gestational diabetes: the offspring follow-up (MiG TOFU): body composition at 2 years of age. Diabetes Care 2011;34(10):2279–84. https://doi.org/10.2337//dc11-660.

40. Morin-Papunen L, Rantala AS, Unkila-Kallio L, et al. Metformin improves pregnancy and live-birth rates in women with polycystic ovary syndrome (PCOS): a multicenter, double-blind, placebo-controlled randomized trial. J Clin Endocrinol Metab 2012;97(5):1492–500. https://doi.org/10.1210/jc.2011-3061.

41. Jovanovic L. Role of diet and insulin treatment of diabetes in pregnancy. Clin Obstet Gynecol 2000;43(1):46–55. https://doi.org/10.1097/00003081-200003000-00005.

42. Hone J, Jovanovic L. Approach to the patient with diabetes during pregnancy. J Clin Endocrinol Metab 2010;95(8):3578–85.

43. California diabetes and pregnancy program. Available at: https://www.cdappsweetsuccess.org/Guidelines-for-Care. April 25, 2021.

44. American Diabetes Association. 10. Cardiovascular disease and risk management: standards of medical care in diabetes—2021. Diabetes Care. 44(Suppl 1): S125-S150.

45. Lundberg GP, Mehta LS. Familial Hypercholesterolemia and pregnancy. American College of Cardiology. Available at: https://www.acc.org/latest-in-cardiology/articles/2018/05/10/13/51/familial-hypercholesterolemia-and-pregnancy. May 22, 2021.

46. American College of Gynecology. Practice bulletin no. 189 summary: nausea and vomiting of pregnancy. Obstet Gynecol 2018;131(1):190–3. https://doi.org/10.1097/AOG.0000000000002450.

47. American Diabetes Association. Management of morning sickness. In: Coustan DR, editor. Medical Management of Pregnancy Complicated by Diabetes. 5th edition. American Diabetes Association; 2013. p. 67–74.

48. Lefevre ML. From preeclampsia: U.S. preventative services task force recommendation statement low-dose aspirin use for the prevention of morbidity and mortality from preeclampsia clinical summary of U.S. preventative services task force recommendation. Ann Intern Med 2014;161(11):819–27.

49. American College of Obstetrics and Gynecology Committee. Low-dose aspirin use during pregnancy. Obstet Gynecol 2018;132(1):e44–51.

50. Moyer VA on behalf of U.S. Preventative Services Task Force. Screening for gestational diabetes mellitus: U.S. task force recommendation statement. Ann Intern Med 2014;160:414–20.

51. Immanuel J, Simmons D. Screening and treatment for early-onset gestational diabetes mellitus: a systematic review and meta-analysis. Curr Diab Rep 2017; 17(11):115. https://doi.org/10.1007/s11892-017-0943-7.

52. Hughes RCE, Moore MP, Gullam JE, et al. An early pregnancy HbA1c >5.9% (41mmol/mol) is optimal for detecting diabetes and identifies women at risk of adverse pregnancy outcomes. Diabetes Care 2014;37:2953–9. https://doi.org/10.2337/dc14-1312.

53. Pons RS, Rockett FC, de Almeida RB, et al. Risk factors for gestational diabetes in a sample of pregnant women diagnosed with the disease. Diabetol Metab Syndr 2015;7(51):A80. https://doi.org/10.1186/1758-5996-7-S1-A80.

54. International Association of Pregnancy Study Groups Consensus Panel. International association of pregnancy study groups recommendations on the diagnosis and classification of hyperglycemia in pregnancy. Diabetes Care 2010;33(3): 676–82.

55. American College of Obstetrics and Gynecology. Practice bulletin no. 190 gestational diabetes. Obstet Gynecol 2018;131(2):e49–64.

56. Hillier TA, Pedula KL, Ogasawara KK, et al. A pragmatic, randomized clinical trial of gestational diabetes screening. N Eng J Med 2021;384(10):895–904. https://doi.org/10.1056/NEJMoa2026028.

57. American associations of diabetes educators practice review gestational diabetes mellitus. Available at: https://www.diabeteseducator.org/docs/default-source/practice/educator-tools/Gestational-Diabetes/gestational-diabetes-mellitus-practice-paper.pdf?sfvrsn=2. May 22, 2021.

58. Leung V, Ragbir-Toolsie K. Perioperative management of patients with diabetes. Health Serv Insights 2017;10:1–5. https://doi.org/10.1177/1178632917735075.

59. American Diabetes Associate. Use of insulin during pregnancy in pre-existing diabetes. In: Coustan DR, editor. Medical management of pregnancy complicated by diabetes. 5th edition. American Diabetes Association; 2013. p. 105–14.

60. Anguzu R, Egede LE, Shour AR, et al. 192-OR association between gestational diabetes and the risk of short interpregnancy intervals. Diabetes 2020;69(Suppl 1). https://doi.org/10.2337/db20-192-OR.

61. Aroda VR, Christophi CA, Edelstein SL, et al, Diabetes Prevention Program Research Group. The effect of lifestyle intervention and metformin on preventing or delaying diabetes among women with and without gestational diabetes: the Diabetes Prevention Program outcomes study 10-year follow-up. J Clin Endocrinol Metab 2015;100:1646–53.

62. Li Z, Cheng Y, Wang D, et al. Incidence rate of type 2 diabetes mellitus after gestational diabetes mellitus: a systematic review and meta- analysis of 170,139 women. J Diabetes Res 2020;2020:3076463.

63. Auvinen AM, Luiro K, Jorkelainen J, et al. Type 1 and type 2 diabetes after gestational diabetes: a 23 year cohort study. Diabetologia 2020;63:2123–8. https://doi.org/10.1007/s00125-020-05215-3.

64. Saravanan P, Diabetes in Pregnancy Working Group, Maternal Medicine Clinical Study Group, Royal College of Obstetricians and Gynaecologists, UK. Gestational diabetes: opportunities for improving maternal and child health. Lancet Diabetes Endocrinol 2020;8(9):793–800. https://doi.org/10.1016/S2213-8587(20)30161-3.

65. Much D, Beyerlein A, RoBbauer M, et al. Beneficial effects of breastfeeding in women with gestational diabetes mellitus. Mol Metab 2014;3:284–92. https://doi.org/10.1016/j.molmet.2014.01.002.

66. American Diabetes Association. Nutrition management of preexisting diabetes during pregnancy. In: Coustan DR, editor. Medical management of pregnancy complicated by diabetes.. 5th edition. American Diabetes Association; 2013. p. 75–98.

Pharmacology—Insulin

Jay H. Shubrook, DO, FAAFP, FACOFP, BC-ADM[a],*,
Kim M. Pfotenhauer, FACOFP[b]

KEYWORDS

- Type 2 diabetes • Insulin • Hyperglycemia • Hypoglycemia

KEY POINTS

- The 3 key elements to know about insulin pharmacokinetics are (1) onset of action, (2) time to peak levels, and (3) duration of action.
- Insulin is the primary treatment of type 1 diabetes. The use of insulin in type 2 diabetes is supported if glucose remains uncontrolled after use of combination oral therapy, glucagon-like peptide-1 receptor agonists, and therapeutic lifestyle changes.
- If the A1c is less than 8.5% start the basal insulin at 0.2 units/kg/d. If the A1c is greater than 8.5%, start at 0.3 unit/kg/d.
- If a person is on an oral secretagogue when starting insulin, consider reducing the dose or stopping the secretagogue if the person is at risk for hypoglycemia.
- To help patients effectively titrate basal insulin inform patients of the expected ceiling dose, parameters to stop titration, and that the starting dose is not the end dose.

INTRODUCTION

Insulin is an important and potent treatment of type 1 and type 2 diabetes. Although many people with type 1 diabetes are treated at specialty centers, the overwhelming majority of people with type 2 diabetes are treated by primary care physicians. Therefore, a working knowledge of insulin and its administration, dosing, and best practices are critical for primary care physicians. Starting people on insulin can be easy, and there are some key best practices to maximize adherence and safety.

BACKGROUND

Insulin is a polypeptide hormone produced and released by the pancreatic β islet cells. In people without diabetes, glucose is normally very tightly controlled by the coordinated secretion of insulin and glucagon as opposing factors to keep glucose in range.[1]

Human endogenous insulin secretion is continuous at baseline to maintain glucose within a narrow window when in a fasting state and while sleeping (basal insulin

[a] Primary Care Department, Touro University California, College of Osteopathic Medicine, Vallejo, CA 94592, USA; [b] Michigan State University, College of Osteopathic Medicine, 965 Wilson Rd, Rm A325, East Lansing, MI 48824-1316, USA
* Corresponding author.
E-mail address: Jshubroo@touro.edu

Prim Care Clin Office Pract 49 (2022) 301–313
https://doi.org/10.1016/j.pop.2021.11.013
0095-4543/22/© 2021 Elsevier Inc. All rights reserved.

primarycare.theclinics.com

secretion). The pancreatic β-cell secretes insulin from vesicles in a pulsatile manner. The amplitude of these pulsatile secretions is based on the ambient glucose level presenting to the pancreas. There is also a diurnal pattern whereby insulin secretion is lowest in the middle of the night and highest first thing in the early morning. In a fasting state, insulin secretion suppresses glycogenolysis and stimulates gluconeogenesis and lipogenesis.[1]

Insulin secretion is also modulated by the intake of nutrients (bolus secretion with food). In response to meal ingestion, insulin secretion is biphasic. There is a rapid first-phase insulin secretion followed by a slower and more sustained second-phase secretion. The incretin system significantly contributes to bolus insulin secretion via the gastrointestinal peptides (glucagon-like peptide-1 [GLP-1] and glucose-dependent insulinotropic polypeptide). These incretin hormones stimulate insulin release and suppress glucagon release from the pancreas, which provides a much larger increase in insulin secretion than ambient glucose levels.[1]

Endogenous insulin is released into the portal venous system, and the liver then removes at least 50% of insulin released. The remainder passes into the systemic circulation where it binds to receptor sites on plasma membranes. This binding leads to a cascade of intracellular reactions that trigger cellular responses such as glucose uptake, glycogen synthesis, and lipogenesis.[1]

Exogenous insulin does not replicate the kinetics of endogenous insulin. Subcutaneously administered exogenous insulin is distributed equally throughout the body (there is no first-pass liver uptake), so the ratio of peripheral insulin to liver insulin is much higher than with endogenous insulin release. This altered ratio is the basis for exogenous insulin pharmacokinetics and the additional side effects of exogenous insulin.

APPROACH

For those with type 1 diabetes, insulin is the primary treatment and is needed to stay alive. Insulin is also the preferred treatment of most people when they are admitted to the hospital and of many women when diabetes complicates pregnancy.[2] Insulin is indicated for people with type 2 diabetes who experience severe hyperglycemia (A1c> 10%) including a fasting glucose level greater than 250 mg/dL indicating glucose toxicity, at the time of surgery to regulate glucose or during an admission to the hospital in which guidelines recommend that oral medications are stopped and insulin is the preferred treatment.[2]

Although insulin can be used in any person with diabetes, it is not the best therapy for everyone. A core pathophysiologic mechanism in type 2 diabetes is insulin resistance. Treating with insulin will contribute further to insulin resistance. Therefore, insulin is best if used at key times in diabetes, started and titrated in a timely manner, and each dose of insulin is targeted to address a specific problem.

THERAPEUTIC OPTIONS

The insulin market has expanded in the last 20 years with more insulin products having been made available for prescription. There are 2 types of human insulin (regular and NPH), 5 U-100 basal insulin analogues (Lantus, Basaglar, Semglee, Levemir, and Tresiba), 6 mealtime insulin analogues (Novolog, Humalog, Apidra, Fiasp, Lyumjev, and Admelog), and 1 inhaled insulin (Afrezza). In addition, there are 4 concentrated insulins (U-500 regular insulin, U-200 Tresiba, U-300 Toujeo, and U-200 Humalog). There are 3 types of premixed insulin product (eg, 70/30 [human and analogue], 75/25 [analogue], 50/50 [analogue]). Each of these insulin products has different pharmacokinetics, onset of action, and duration of action. Thus, optimizing effectiveness and ensuring safety of insulin therapy involves many factors for clinicians to consider (**Table 1**).

INSULIN PHYSIOLOGY

Endogenous insulin is active when it is in its monomeric form; this is important, as keeping insulin in the monomeric form or delaying breakdown into monomers can be used to change the onset and duration of insulin. The body can buffer insulin with zinc, which allows it to form dimers and hexamers. In turn, these act as stabilizers to insulin, particularly in β-cell vesicles.

When insulin is injected into the subcutaneous tissue, it is usually in hexameric form, which later dissociates into monomers. The rate of dissociation from hexamers and dimers to monomers is responsible for the onset and duration of action (time action profiles) of the different insulin preparations. In commercially available insulins, the use of a zinc buffer can help increase the stability and duration of action of regular insulin (R) and neutral protamine hagedorn (NPH). To further the duration of NPH, a phosphate buffer is used, and the molecule is protaminated.

The time action profiles of the analogue insulins start with an amino acid substitution to change the kinetics, either to keep insulin as a monomer or to extend time action by keeping insulin molecules in dimers and hexamers. Further, glargine uses an acidic pH to help provide longer stability. Detemir and degludec are also bound to a free fatty acid, which then binds to albumin to prolong duration of action. Degludec has the longest duration of action; this is made possible by its ability to form chains of hexamers that slow the dissociation into monomers and allow for a longer duration of action.

The onset of action of an insulin (eg, rapid, fast, intermediate) can provide a window for dosing in relation to food. The time to peak levels of an insulin will provide information about when a person is most likely to drop their serum glucose levels. The duration of action will provide insight into when insulin can be safely dosed again (**Table 2**).

Rapid-Acting Insulins

There are 7 Food and Drug Administration–approved rapid-acting insulin analogues available in the United States today: glulisine, lispro, biosimilar lispro, aspart, fast-acting aspart, insulin lispro-aabb, and inhaled insulin Technosphere. Most are provided by subcutaneous injection, but inhaled insulin Technosphere is administered by oral inhalation. All of the injectables of these are clear, colorless solutions. Timing of meals and monitoring for hypoglycemia are important with rapid-acting insulins.

All of the aforementioned insulins are intended to be taken with a meal and should be dosed 15 to 30 minutes before a meal to allow insulin absorption and onset to match the absorption of food. When these 2 parts are well-timed, the risk of postmeal hypoglycemia and hyperglycemia is reduced.[2] When these insulins are used to treat hyperglycemia outside of mealtime care should be taken to ensure that the additional dose of insulin does not overlap with mealtime dosing and that the scale is individually calculated based on weight and insulin sensitivity.

Short-Acting Insulin

Regular insulin (Humulin R, Novulin R, ReliOn R) is a short-acting human insulin produced using recombinant DNA techniques. Its form is a clear, soluble crystalline zinc solution. This insulin molecule will aggregate in dimers and hexamers when administered in high concentrations, slowing absorption. Regular insulin is normally administered 30 to 45 minutes before a meal and tends to last longer than rapid-acting insulins, anywhere from 4 to 12 hours—the duration of action is dose dependent.[8,33]

Table 1
Landscape of human and analogue insulins

Insulin	Analogue	Analogue Brand Name	Human	Human Insulin Brand Name
Ultra-rapid	Insulin Aspart Insulin Lispro-aabb	Fiasp Lyumjev	Inhaled human insulin —	Afrezza —
Rapid	Aspart Biosimilar Lispro Glulisine Lispro	NovoLOG Admelog Apidra HumaLOG	—	—
Fast	—	—	Regular	HumuLIN R NovoLIN R ReliOn[a] R
Intermediate	—	—	NPH	HumuLIN NPH NovoLIN R ReliOn[a] R
Long-acting	Detemir Glargine	Levemir Lantus Basaglar Semglee	—	—
Ultra-longacting	Degludec	Tresiba	—	—
Premixed insulin combinations	Aspart/Pegylated Apart Lispro/Peglyated Lispro	NovoLOG 70/30 HumaLOG 75/25 Humalog 50/50	Regular/NPH	HumuLIN 70/30 NovoLIN 70/30 ReliOn[a] 70/30
Concentrated Insulin	Degludec U200 Glargine U300 Lispro U200	Tresiba Toujeo HumaLOG	Regular U500	HumuLIN U500
—	—	—	—	—

[a] ReliOn is only available at Walmart for cash-paying patients.

Data from Young CY, Dugan J, Kuang HY et al. Insulin Therapy for Type 2 Diabetes: Social, Psychological, and Clinical Factors. Primary Care Reports January 2019. 25:1:1 to 12.

Table 2
Pharmacokinetic profiles of currently available human insulins and insulin analogues

Insulin	Brand Name/ Manufacturer	Available as	Species Source	Conc.	Time of Action (h)		
					Onset	Peak Effect	Duration
Glulisine[13]	Apidra/Sanofi[3]	Vial/Solostar pens	Human analogue	U100	0.2–0.5	1.6–2.8	3–4
Lispro[14]	HumaLOG[34] Eli Lilly	Vials/pens	Human analogue	U100	0.25–0.5	0.5–2.5	≤ 5
Aspart[15]	NovoLOG Novonordisk[4]	Vial/flexpens	Human analogue	U100	0.2–0.3	1–3	3–5
Insulin Aspart[16]	FIASP Novonordisk[5]	Vials/pens	Human analogue	U100	0.12	1–3	3–5
Biosimilar Lispro[17]	Admelog Sanofi[6]	Pens	Human biosimilar	U100	0.25–0.5	0.5–2.5	≤ 5
Insulin Lispro-aabc[18]	Lyumjev Eli Lilly[7]	Vials/pens	Human analogue	U100			
Regular[19,20]	HumuLIN R[33] NovoLIN R[8] Eli Lilly, Novonordisk	Vials/pens	human	U100	0.5	2.5–5	4–12
NPH[21,22]	HumuLIN N[9] NovoLIN N[10] Eli Lilly, Novonordisk	Vials/pens	Human	U100	1–2	4–12	14–24
70 NPH 30 Regular[23,24]	HumuLIN 70/30[11] NovoLIN 70/30[12] Eli Lilly, Novonordisk	Vials/pens	Human	U100	0.5	Regular 0.8–2 NPH 6–10	18–24
50 lispro protamine 50 lispro[25]	HumaLOG Mix 50/50[13]	Vials/pens	Human analogue	U100	0.25–0.5	0.8–4.8	14–24
75 lispro protamined 25 lispro[26]	HumaLOG Mix	Vials/pens	Human analogue	U100	0.25–0.5	1–6.5	14–24

(continued on next page)

Table 2
(continued)

Insulin	Brand Name/Manufacturer	Available as	Species Source	Conc.	Time of Action (h)		
					Onset	Peak Effect	Duration
70 aspart protamined 30 aspart[27]	75/25[14] Eli Lilly / NovoLOG Mix 70/30[15] Novonordisk	Vials/flexpens	Human analogue	U100	0.15–0.3	1–4	18–24
70 degludec/30 aspart[28]	Ryzodec Novonordisk[16]	Pens	Human analogue	U100	0.12–0.25	1–2	>25
Detemir[29]	Levemir Novonordisk[17]	Vials/flexpens	Human analogue	U100	3–4	3–9	6–23
Glargine[30]	Lantus Sanofi[18] Semglee[20]	Vials/Solostar pens Vials/pens	Human analogue	U100	3–4	None	Mean 24
Biosimilar Glargine[31]	Basaglar Eli Lilly[19]	Pens	Human biosimiliar	U100	3–4	none	Mean 24
Degludec[32]	Tresiba Novonordisk[21]	Pens	Human analogue	U100	1	none	42
Regular[33]	HumuLIN R U500 Eli Lilly[22]	Pens/vials	Human	U500	0.5	2.5–5	Up to 24
Lispro[34]	Humalog U200 Eli Lilly[23]	Pens	Human analogue	U200	0.25–0.5	0.5–2.5	≤5
Glargine[35]	Toujeo[35] Sanofi	Pens	Human analogue	U300	6	None	24
Degludec[32]	Tresiba Novonordisk[21]	Pens	Human analogue	U200	1	None	42

Rapid   Short   Intermediate   Long   Intermediate/Short-Acting Mixed   Intermediate/Rapid-Acting Mixed   Concentrated (Variable Duration)

Data from Young CY, Dugan J, Kuang HY et al. Insulin Therapy for Type 2 Diabetes: Social, Psychological, and Clinical Factors. Primary Care Reports January 2019.

Regular insulin can be given subcutaneously. It is also particularly useful as an intravenous infusion and is frequently used in hyperglycemic crises such as diabetic ketoacidosis and hyperglycemic hyperosmolar nonketosis syndrome. In the hospital setting regular insulin is the preferred intravenous insulin, as it is inexpensive and all exogenous insulins quickly dissociate into monomers when given intravenously.

Intermediate-Acting Insulin

NPH (isophane) is a cloudy insulin suspension that contains insulin and protamine. The addition of protamine creates a longer duration of action. When administered, enzymes slowly break down the protamine to allow for the slow absorption of insulin. NPH absorption is often variable, having an onset from 1 to 5 hours and duration of action from 4 to 12 hours. Insulin NPH is available as HumuLIN N (Lilly) or NovoLIN N (Novo Nordisk).[9,10] In the clinical setting NPH is typically given one meal in advance (eg, before breakfast to cover lunch or before dinner to cover a bedtime snack) or as 2 to 3 doses per day to serve as a basal insulin.

PRE-MIXED INSULINS

Premixed insulins were developed to improve convenience for patients by reducing dosing frequency. There are human insulin mixes and rapid analogue insulin mixes. The human premixed insulin uses R insulin mixed with NPH. The premixed analogue insulins use rapid-acting insulin analogue and a protaminated version of the rapid-acting analogue. The time to onset, peak, and duration are dictated by the short-acting component. Patients should be instructed on the differences between these insulin mixes (regular vs analog-based). Premixed insulins are named by the percentage of each component insulin/analogue, with the longer-acting insulin first. To improve safety and clarity the last 3 letters of premixed insulins are capitalized to better identify human from analogue insulins and prevent accidental switches.

Human insulin NPH/regular insulin mix is commercially available in 2 brands: HumuLIN 70/30 or NovoLIN N 70/30 (70% NPH and 30% regular).[11,12] The 70/30 mix is a cloudy suspension (NPH is cloudy). For the human insulin mix the onset is around 30 to 45 minutes with a peak effect in 4 to 12 hours. This insulin is typically dosed 2 to 3 times per day with prebreakfast and predinner dosing; this is convenient for patients who want to limit the number of injections. Responses to this insulin, although, can be less reliable dose to dose than nonmixed insulins. Regular insulin can precipitate out in the NPH insulin suspension, which can contribute to day-to-day variability in the action profiles of the insulin.

Other mixed insulins available include rapid-acting analogue insulin and protaminated rapid-acting analogue insulin. The protaminated rapid-acting analogue will delay absorption and give a prolonged effect. The HumaLOG 75/25 and NovoLOG 70/30 mixes have a more rapid onset of action and a shorter peak effect[14,15]; this allows them to be dosed immediately before mealtime, which may result in more reliable clinical effects and reduced postmeal hypoglycemia. Premixed insulins are ideal for people who need both basal and mealtime insulin coverage but want to limit the number of injections per day. People taking premixed insulin will want to maintain a regular schedule of meals times and carbohydrate content to maximize benefit and minimize risk.

LONG-ACTING ANALOG (BASAL) INSULINS

The introduction of a steady, long-acting insulin closely mimics the basal rate of endogenous insulin. These agents alone have a lower risk of hypoglycemia (compared with NPH) due to the lack of a peak response and the continuous release of low levels of insulin. These insulins are typically given once daily independent of meals.

Insulin glargine is a long-acting analogue of human insulin. The insulin structure is modified by attaching 2 arginine amino acids to the terminal end of the B chain and changing asparagine to glycine at the terminal end of the A chain. These modifications produce a clear, colorless solution that is soluble in acid and forms a precipitate on subcutaneous injection. This precipitate dissolves slowly, creating a continuous, steady release of insulin. Because of this mechanism, insulin glargine has no defined peak. Glargine is injected subcutaneously once daily and should not be administered intravenously or intramuscularly.[19] Given that glargine has an acidic pH, it should not be mixed with other insulins. Some patients report a burning sensation at the injection site as a result of the acidic pH, but this is not an indicator of any adverse effect. There are 3 formulations of glargine U100 (Lantus, Basaglar, and Semglee, and U300 glargine -Tuojeo)[18–20,35]

Insulin detemir (Levemir) is a clear, colorless, long-acting human analogue insulin. The threonine on the terminal end of the B chain is dropped and C-14 fatty acid chain is attached to the B29 lysine. When injected, the fatty acid chain reversibly binds detemir to albumin, which slows each step of absorption from the subcutaneous tissue to the cell. The onset of action is generally 1 to 2 hours. Insulin detemir can be given once daily, administered subcutaneously.[17]

Insulin degludec (Tresiba) has a duration of 42 hours. This protracted duration of action is due to its ability to form not only hexamers but also chains of hexamers. It is available in both U100 and U200 concentrations.[21]

All basal insulins have similar efficacy. The ideal person to take a basal insulin analogue is someone completely insulin deficient (type 1 diabetes), someone at high risk for hypoglycemia (day or nighttime), or someone with a highly variable schedule making a consistent dosing difficult. One exception is that when switching from U100 glargine to U300 glargine the dose may need to be increased by about 18% for the same efficacy.[21]

CONCENTRATED INSULINS

With the global pandemic of obesity, we see much higher rates of diabetes. Those who are obese and have type 2 diabetes typically need more insulin for a therapeutic effect, which often means very large doses of daily insulin (200–300 units per day). Once a person needs more than 300 units of insulin per day, the number of injections increases, and the pharmacokinetics of the insulin can be less consistent due to potential depot effects at the injection site. Concentrated insulins are a potential solution to this challenge. Another potential solution is to use other complimentary therapies (including lifestyle and other medications) that limit the insulin burden in those with type 2 diabetes and substantial insulin resistance (**Fig. 1**).

GUIDELINES FOR BEST PRACTICES IN INSULIN USE

Insulin is the primary treatment of type 1 diabetes, and all patients with type 1 need to have strong skills in insulin management. Current guidelines by the American Diabetes Association and American Association of Clinical Endocrinologists support the use of insulin in type 2 diabetes if glucose remains uncontrolled after use of combination oral therapy, GLP-1 receptor agonists, and therapeutic lifestyle changes.[2,25] In addition, insulin may also be the preferred initial treatment of patients who present with severe hyperglycemia; this includes those with a fasting glucose greater than 250 mg/dL,

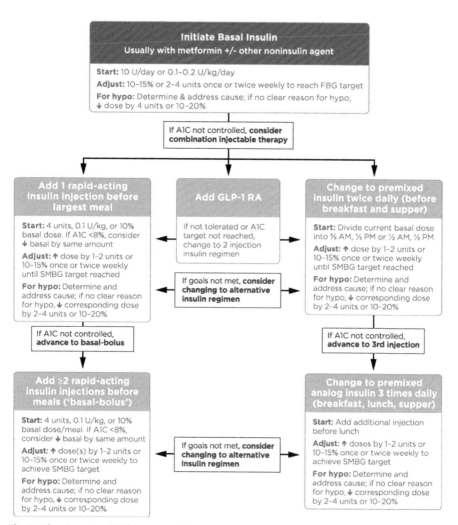

Fig. 1. The American Diabetes Association recommendations for initiating injectable therapies. (Reprinted with permission from The American Diabetes Association. Copyright 2021 by the American Diabetes Association.)

HgA1c greater than 10%, or acute symptoms of insulin deficiency including polyuria, polydipsia, and weight loss.

Insulin may be needed as part of the treatment plan for people with type 2 diabetes. For these patients, starting insulin usually means starting a basal insulin, for example, NPH, glargine, detemir, and degludec. Basal insulins allow for suppression of hepatic glucose production overnight and can help normalize morning blood glucose. Therefore, controlling fasting glucose is a logical first step. By removing glucose toxicity, the remaining functioning β cells are better able to address prandial hyperglycemia.

Any medication that also increases secretion of insulin should be examined. These include the sulfonylureas and the metaglinides. Sulfonylureas and metaglinides should be stopped if the patient is starting on meal-time insulin, as this combination substantially increases the risk of hypoglycemia.

Most medications can be safely used with insulin. Metformin should be continued in most patients as long as possible. The dose of thiazolidinediones should be lowered if the patient is already having problems with weight gain or edema. The dipeptidyl-peptidase 4 inhibitors can be safely taken with insulin and are often complementary to basal insulin. No dose adjustment is needed when starting insulin. GLP-1 receptor agonists can be safely used with insulin. In fact, this is a potent combination, and many people who start a GLP-1 RA after insulin can reduce the insulin dose and maintain improved control. The SGLT-2 inhibitors can also be used safely with basal insulin. Often these meds will also help to reduce the need for insulin.

Teaching an injection: it is not common for patients to be excited or even comfortable with injecting insulin. We can improve adherence and longevity of insulin use by equipping patients with the knowledge to safely inject insulin. Key steps to teaching insulin administration include teaching the person how to use the device (insulin syringe, or insulin pen), making sure the first injection is supervised (in the office or with a staff member or educator), providing expected benefits, and giving warnings of when the patient should contact the office.

Injection technique: insulin is intended to be injected into the subcutaneous tissue. There are many areas available for insulin injections in most patients. A chart of potential insulin injection sites is shown later. With any injectable treatment, it is important to rotate sites so none of the sites become scarred (leading to impaired absorption of insulin) (**Fig. 2**).

Insulin titration: most insulin doses will need to be titrated to obtain the desired treatment effect. There is good evidence that helping patients titrate their own insulin dosing is not only safe but also effective.[5,6] Common basal insulin titrations include the following, each using a fasting glucose as the target trying to achieve: (1) increasing the dose by 1 unit daily; (2) increasing by 2 to 4 units 2 times per week; (3) increasing 5 to 7 units weekly.[7] A careful look at the math shows that each of these regimens are providing a similar increase in insulin every week.

Many patients will be nervous about increasing the dose of insulin for fear of taking too much and dropping low. There are some best practices to help the patient stay on course for titration:

1. Please let the patient know the starting dose is expected to be less than needed for full effect.
2. Let the patient know what is the ceiling dose for this titration schedule (we typically use 0.5 units/kg).
3. Provide parameters when the patient should stop titrating—when they achieve the target fasting glucose, when they reach the ceiling dose (0.5 units/kg), or anytime they experience hypoglycemia.

By providing a ceiling dose patients will understand that you know they will need more insulin than they started with; this also provides a stopping point at which they should reach out and get advice.

Devices: insulin can be delivered by vial and syringe, prefilled insulin pen, and continuous insulin secretion by insulin pump. It is often helpful for the health care provider to know what each of the devices look like, as patients may be more familiar with pen appearance than insulin name. For example, "I take the gray pen at night and the pen with orange before my meals." A complete index of all devices is published annually in Diabetes Spectrum.[32]

Checking for scar tissue: any person can develop scar tissue when taking repeated injections. Scar tissue can present as lipohypertrophy (raised and hard) or lipoatrophy

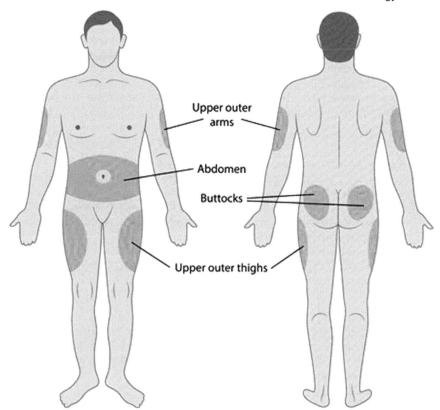

Fig. 2. Insulin injections sites. (*From* Insulin injection sites. National Health Service UK- diabetes resources. Available at: https://diabetesmyway.nhs.uk/resources/internal/why-is-my-blood-glucose-high/. Accessed 9/27/21.)

(subcutaneous fat breakdown or dimpling). Proper insulin injection technique and rotation of injection sites can substantially reduce this risk.

Hypoglycemia: hypoglycemia is one of the most feared side effects of insulin injection. It is important to make sure all patients on insulin are educated on the common signs and symptoms of hypoglycemia, learn how to treat hypoglycemia with the rule of 15s, and have a prescription for glucagon to treat severe hypoglycemia. At each visit it is very helpful to ask the patient if they have had any hypoglycemic episodes, what they felt, and how they treated them.

Starting/adjusting meal time insulin: once a patient has the fasting glucose at or near target, the attention then can be moved to see if there is adequate mealtime coverage. For people with type 2 diabetes the dose started is typically 4 units per meal or 10% to 20% of the total basal insulin dose. It is important to remind people who are taking insulin that dosing before meals is much safer than during or after meals, and knowledge of the onset of each type of insulin can provide a guide for this timing.

Titration of mealtime insulin can be challenging. Many people alter the timing and the nutrient content of their meals, and this could affect insulin dosing. Although carbohydrate counting is commonly used in type 1 diabetes, it is not always recommended in type 2 diabetes due to the substantial active calculations and limited benefits in many people with type 2 diabetes. Instead, the recommendation is to consider relative carbohydrate consistency at meals to get a consistent response from fixed insulin dosing.

Starting/adjusting premixed insulin: premixed insulin is often used to reduce the number of injections a person has to take. This insulin can contribute to cost savings but does require some level of consistency in daily eating schedule and carbohydrate consistency at meals. Strong knowledge of insulin kinetics is needed to safely and effectively use these insulins. Timing of doses is based on the number of meals eaten, timing, and spacing of the meals.

COST OF INSULINS

The cost of insulin has become a significant clinical and public health issue. Although there are many new expensive insulin products, even the costs of many of the older insulins have skyrocketed. These costs have contributed to substantial hardships for many patients, especially those responsible for some or all the price of their medications.

Potential responses have included patients not taking insulin as prescribed, patients relying on samples when they are not covered or underinsured, or just not filling the insulin at all. It has been estimated that 1 in 4 Americans on insulin ration their insulin because of the cost[24]; this has resulted in professional organizations and health care systems taking action to limit the cost of insulin in the United States.[2]

SUMMARY

Although insulin is an important treatment of type 1 diabetes, judicious use in type 2 diabetes should be considered. The primary care physician should be knowledgeable about the decision for use, initiation of treatment and titration as well as common pitfalls such as hypoglycemia and cost.

CLINICS CARE POINTS

- The 3 key elements to know about insulin pharmacokinetics are (1) onset of action, (2) time to peak levels, and (3) duration of action.
- If the A1c is less than 8.5% start the basal insulin at 0.2 units/kg/day—if the A1c is greater than 8.5% start at 0.3 unit/kg/d.
- If a person is on an oral secretagogue when starting insulin, consider reducing the dose or stopping the secretagogue if the person is at risk for hypoglycemia.
- To help patients effectively titrate basal insulin dose please provide this information: starting dose will need to be increased, expected ceiling dose, and parameters to stop titration.

REFERENCES

1. Jameson JL, DeGroot LJ, De Kretser DM, et al. Endocrinology Adult and Pediatric. 7th edition. Saunder Co; 2016. p. 544–55. Chapter 32.
2. American Diabetes Association Standards of Medical Care in Diabetes 2021. Available at: https://care.diabetesjournals.org/content/44/Supplement_1_1. Accessed September 27 2021.
3. Apidra (insulin glulisine). Package insert. Bridgewater, (NJ): Sanofi; 2019.
4. Novolog (insulin aspart). Package insert. Plainsboro, (NJ): Novo Nordisk; 2021.
5. FIASP (Inulin aspart). Package insert. Plainsboro, (NJ): Novo Nordisk; 2019.
6. Admelog (Biosimilar lispro). Package insert. Bridgewater, (NJ): Sanofi; 2019.
7. Lyumjev (Insluin lispro-aabc). Package insert. Indianapolis: Lilly USA, LLC; 2021.
8. NovoLIN R. (Regular insulin). Package insert. Princeton, (NJ): Novo Nordisk; 2012.

9. HumuLIN N. (NPH). Package insert. Indianapolis: Lilly USA, LLC; 2019.
10. NovoLIN N. (NPH). Package insert. Princeton, (NJ): Novo Nordisk; 2012.
11. HumuLIN 70/30. Package insert. Indianapolis: Lilly USA, LLC; 2019.
12. NovoLIN 70/30. Package insert. Plainsboro, (NJ): Novo Nordisk; 2019.
13. HumaLOG mix 50/50. Package insert. Indianapolis: Lilly USA, LLC; 2015.
14. HumaLOG Mix 75/25 (75 lispro protamine d/25 lispro). Package Insert. Indianapolis: Lilly USA, LLC; 2019.
15. NovoLOG mix 70/30. Package insert. Princeton, (NJ): Novo Nordisk; 2007.
16. Ryzodeg 70/30 (insulin degludec and insulin aspart). Package Insert. Plainsboro (NJ): Novo Nordisk; 2019.
17. Levemir (insulin detemir). Package insert. Plainsboro, (NJ): Novo Nordisk; 2020.
18. Lantus (insulin glargine). Package insert. Bridgewater, (NJ): Sanofi; 2019.
19. Basaglar (biosimilar insulin glargine). Package Insert. Indianapolis: Lilly USA, LLC; 2021.
20. Semglee (insulin glargine) Package insert. Mylan Pharmaceuticals. Morgantown WV; 2020.
21. Tresiba (insulin degludec). Package Insert. Plainsboro, (NJ): Novo Nordisk; 2019.
22. HumuLIN R U-500 (regular). Indianapolis: Lilly USA, LLC; 2019.
23. HumaLOG U-200 (insulin lispro). Indianapolis: Lilly USA, LLC; 2019.
24. Crowley MJ, Maciejewski ML. Revisiting NPH insulin for type 2 diabetes: is a step back the path. JAMA 2018;320(1):38–9.
25. AACE/ACE Consensus Statement on treatment of hyperglycemia. Available at: https://pro.aace.com/pdfs/diabetes/algorithm-exec-summary.pdf.   Accessed September 27 2021.
26. Insulin injection sites. National Health Service UK- diabetes resources. Available at: https://diabetesmyway.nhs.uk/resources/internal/why-is-my-blood-glucose-high/. Accessed September 27 2021.
27. Harris SB, Yale JF, Berard L, et al. Does a patient-managed insulin intensification strategy with insulin glargine and insulin glulisine provide similar glycemic control as a physician-managed strategy? Results of the START (Self-Titration with Apidra to Reach Target) study: a randomized noninferiority trial. Diabetes Care 2014;37:604–10.
28. Oyer DS, Shepherd MD, Coulter FC, et al. A1c control in a primary care setting: self-titrating an insulin analog pre-mix (INITIATEplus Trial). Am J Med 2009;122: 1043–9.
29. Davies M, Storms F, Shutler S, et al. Improvement of glycemic control in subjects with poorly controlled type 2 diabetes: comparison of two treatment algorithms using insulin glargine. Diabetes Care 2005;28:1282–8.
30. Meneghini L, Koenen C, Weng W, et al. The usage of a simplified self-titration dosing guideline (303 Algorithm) for insulin detemir in patients with type 2 diabetes: results of the randomized, controlled PREDICTIVE™ 303 study. Diabetes Obes Metab 2007;9:902–13.
31. Yale JF, Harris SB, Berard L, et al. A pragmatic self-titration 1 unit/day (INSIGHT) algorithm for insulin glargine 300 U/mL (GLA-300) (Abstract). Diabetes 2016; 65(Suppl. 1A):93. LB [Google Scholar].
32. ADA Consumer Guide. Available at: http://archives.diabetesforecast.org/2019/ 02-mar-apr/consumer-guide-2019.html. Accessed September 27 2021.
33. HumuLIN R. (Regular insulin). Package insert. Indianapolis: Lilly USA, LLC; 2019.
34. HumaLOG (insulin lispro). Package insert. Eli Lilly and Company; 2020.
35. Toujeo. (insulin glargine). Package insert. Bridgewater, NJ: Sanofi; 2015.

Pharmacology
Non-Insulin Agents

Heather O'Brien, PharmD, CPP[a],*,
Catherine Travis, PharmD, BCACP, CPP[b]

KEYWORDS

- Non-insulin • Diabetes pharmacology • Diabetes treatment • Type 2 diabetes

KEY POINTS

- Several noninsulin agent classes have become first-line agents for adults with uncontrolled type-2 diabetes
- Studies have indicated that several noninsulin agents offer cardiovascular and renal protection
- Metformin remains the first line in the treatment of type 2 diabetes
- Patient specific factors may help guide decision making for the treatment of type 2 diabetes

PHARMACOLOGY: NONINSULIN AGENTS
Background

While the history and development of diabetes medication dates back to the 1920s with Dr Frederick Banting and his team developing the first commercially available insulin, manufacturing of noninsulin products has a much shorter timeline.[1] Since the early 1900s, additional medication classes have been identified, formulated, and prescribed—allowing for the deescalation of insulin therapy and improved patient outcomes. From sulfonylureas being prescribed in the 1930s to the advent of sodium–glucose cotransporter 2 inhibitors (SGLT2s), in 2013, advances continue to promote not only improved diabetes control but also renal and cardiovascular benefits.[2]

This article will draw on recent studies and guidelines to direct up-to-date patient care. The 2021 American Diabetes Association (ADA) Guidelines call for a patient-centered approach to care based on a multitude of factors including hemoglobin A1c, concomitant disease states, cost, etc. As such, while achieving a target A1c is ideal, ensuring patient adherence and acceptance of the plan guides treatment decisions. This article will first introduce the different drug classes and their individual benefits before summarizing how each fits into the treatment algorithm.

[a] Southern Regional Area Health Education Center, 1601 Owen Drive, Fayetteville, NC 28304, USA; [b] Cone Health, 1200 North Elm St, Greensboro, NC 27401, USA
* Corresponding author.
E-mail address: heather.obrien@sr-ahec.org

Prim Care Clin Office Pract 49 (2022) 315–326
https://doi.org/10.1016/j.pop.2021.11.010
primarycare.theclinics.com

Table 1 provides a list of common abbreviations that will be used throughout this article.

DRUG CLASSES
Metformin

Metformin should generally be considered first-line therapy for type 2 diabetes (T2DM), given affordability, low hypoglycemic potential, and positive cardiovascular benefit.[2,3] Metformin works by decreasing hepatic gluconeogenesis and increasing insulin sensitivity in peripheral tissues.[4] It is an effective agent, lowering A1c by 1.0% to 1.5%. Metformin is generally well tolerated, with the most common side effects being gastrointestinal upset, including bloating, abdominal discomfort, and diarrhea. These side effects may be lessened by a slow initial titration. Additionally, changing from immediate-release to extended-release formulations may also improve tolerance.

The drug is excreted renally, and high circulating levels of drug have been rarely associated with lactic acidosis. Therefore, most recent labeling recommendations note to avoid use in patients with eGFR less than 30 mL/min. Some experts recommend considering a dose reduction if eGFR falls to less than 45 mL/min while on therapy and avoiding initiation altogether with eGFR less than 45.[5] Metformin use has also been found to be associated with Vitamin B12 deficiency.[6]

In practice, metformin should be started in patients when they are first diagnosed with diabetes, excepting patients with kidney disease as discussed above. Once titrated to a maximally tolerated dose, metformin should not be removed from therapy, even when insulin or other agents have been initiated.[2] Discontinuation occurs when the medication is contraindicated or poorly tolerated by the patient.

Notably, metformin is now recommended for use in patients with a diagnosis of prediabetes, as well as polycystic ovarian syndrome (PCOS) which can be a precursor for insulin resistance and diabetes.[7,8]

Sodium– Glucose Cotransporter 2 Inhibitors

Sodium–glucose cotransporter 2 inhibitors (SGLT2i) have quickly become a highly recommended medication class in the treatment of Type 2 diabetes. This class is a versatile option for the treatment of diabetes, as well as heart failure and chronic kidney disease. SGLT2i inhibit glucose reabsorption in the renal tubules, resulting in glucosuria that reduces A1c by 0.5% to 1.0%.[9] SGLT2i are associated with an increased

Table 1 Common abbreviations	
Description:	**Abbreviation**
Type 2 Diabetes	T2DM
American Diabetes Association	ADA
Sodium glucose cotransporter 2 inhibitors	SGLT-2i
Glucagon-like peptide-1 receptor agonist	GLP1
Dipeptidyl-peptidase inhibitors	DPP4
Sulfonylurea	SU
Gastrointestinal	GI
Cardiovascular Outcome Trials	CVOT
Subcutaneous	Subq
MACE	Major Adverse Cardiac Events

risk of mycotic genitourinary infections. Increased glucosuria can be associated with an increased risk of volume depletion and dehydration, making it important to counsel patients to stay appropriately hydrated while on therapy.[5] Postmarketing reports have shown an association with euglycemic diabetic ketoacidosis, prompting FDA recommendations to hold this class of medications before surgery.[10] This medication is associated with weight loss, though this is generally thought to be related to fluid. **Table 2** shows a comparison of the different medications within the SGLT2i class.

In concordance with the 2008 FDA recommendation regarding the study of new diabetes medications and their effect on cardiovascular events and mortality, each medication in the SGLT2i (as well as GLP-1 and DPP4) class has undergone cardiovascular outcomes trials (CVOTs) investigating potential risk versus benefit in an intention-to-treat model.[11] The agents in the SGLT2i class have been found to have significant benefits in additional disease states, prompting recent labeling expansions. Empagliflozin and canagliflozin demonstrated significant reductions in a cardiovascular composite outcome (myocardial infarction, stroke, and cardiovascular death) compared with placebo, therefore prompting an additional indication to reduce the risk of cardiovascular death in diabetes.[12,13] The DAPA-HF and EMPEROR-reduced trials demonstrated significant reductions in a composite outcome of heart failure hospitalizations and cardiovascular death compared with placebo for dapagliflozin and empagliflozin, respectively.[14,15] These trials were conducted in patients with and without diabetes at baseline. In May of 2020, dapagliflozin labeling was updated to include an indication to reduce the risk of heart failure hospitalizations in patients with heart failure with reduced ejection fraction (regardless of diabetes diagnosis) and New York Heart Association Class II-IV.[16] This drug class also has benefits in reducing the progression of chronic kidney disease. Despite initial hesitation for use in patients with reduced kidney function, secondary outcomes from the previous cardiovascular outcomes trials indicated a possible reduction in the progression of nephropathy. The CREDENCE trial in patients with type 2 diabetes found that canagliflozin reduced the risk of a primary composite outcome of end-stage kidney disease, doubling of serum creatine, or death from renal causes versus placebo.[17] The DAPA-CKD trial enrolled patients with and without diabetes, and found a significant reduction in a primary composite outcome of a sustained decline in the estimated GFR of at least 50%, end-stage kidney disease, or death from renal causes, prompting an addition of renal benefit labeling to dapagliflozin in April 2020.[18]

Glucagon-Like Peptide-1 Receptor Agonists

Much like SGLT2i, the glucagon-like peptide-1 (GLP-1) receptor agonists have become a mainstay in the treatment of T2DM. Offering additional benefits beyond A1c lowering, the GLP-1 class works to improve diabetes by decreasing hepatic glucose production, stimulating pancreatic insulin release, and slowing gastric emptying. Slowing of the gastrointestinal tract results in increased satiety and can result in weight loss.[19,20] Both liraglutide and semaglutide have obtained FDA-approved indications for use in weight loss and are trademarked as Saxenda and Wegovy, respectively.[21,22] Classwide, these medications can result in nausea and vomiting, which typically resolves within 1 to 2 weeks after starting the medication.[23] Once tolerated and titrated to a therapeutically effective dose, these medications work on postprandial blood glucose and can lower A1c by an average of 1% to 1.5%.[24] When first released, these medications were formulated as daily or weekly injections. However, with the release of oral semaglutide (Rybelsus) in September 2019, patients now have the opportunity to receive the benefits of a GLP-1 without the need for injections. Oral semaglutide was found to be noninferior to liraglutide in A1c reduction

Table 2			
SGLT2 comparison table			
Brand Name	Generic Name	Dosing Schedule	Additional Comments
Invokana	Canagliflozin	100 and 300 mg daily Do not initiate therapy in patients with eGFR <30	A1c Reduction: 0.77%-1.03% Weight loss: 4.8–7.3 lb
Farxiga	Dapagliflozin	5mg and 10 mg daily Do not use in patients with eGFR <25	A1c reduction: 0.8%–0.9% Weight loss: 3.0–4.4 lb FDA approval for use in Heart Failure
Jardiance	Empagliflozin	10 mg and 25 mg once daily Do not use in patients with eGFR <30	A1c reduction: 0.7%–0.8% Weight loss: 5.5–6.2 lb FDA approval for use in Heart Failure
Steglatro	Ertugliflozin	5 and 15 mg once daily Do not use in patients with eGFR <30	A1c reduction: 0.7%–0.8% Weight loss: 4.4–4.6 lb

and superior in weight loss after 26 weeks.[25] **Table 3** shows a comparison of the different medications within the GLP-1 class.

As discussed above, each medication in the GLP-1 class has undergone CVOTs investigating potential risk versus benefit in an intention-to-treat model. No study showed inherent risk in CV outcomes; however, liraglutide, semaglutide (injection only), and dulaglutide have all shown noninferiority to placebo.[26] Of these trials, the *LEADER* (liraglutide), *SUSTAIN-6 (*semaglutide), and *REWIND* (dulaglutide) trials studied patients who either had a history of CV disease or risk factors for CV disease. *LEADER, HARMONY, and REWIND* all demonstrated superiority in cardiovascular outcomes compared with placebo, with *REWIND* studying primarily patients without established CV disease at baseline. *SUSTAIN-6* did not prespecify superiority. The most recent CVOT, *Pioneer 6,* looking at oral semaglutide was a noninferiority trial showing a similar hazard ratio (0.79 vs 0.74) to the injectable semaglutide.[27–33]

While no studies have been published exploring the possible renal protective benefits of GLP-1s as a primary outcome, the previous CVOT did investigate renal outcomes as secondary endpoints. *LEADER, SUSTAIN-6, and REWIND* all demonstrated a possible decrease in the development of new-onset macroalbuminuria, but no significant reductions were found when looking at the reduction of eGFR than placebo.[34]

Dipeptidyl Peptidase 4 Inhibitors

Similar to the GLP-1 class, dipeptidyl peptidase 4 (DPP4) inhibitors work on the incretin hormone system. By preventing the enzyme DPP4 from breaking down GLP-1 and glucose-dependent insulinotropic polypeptide (GIP), these agents help stimulate pancreatic beta cells to release insulin, while decreasing the secretion of glucagon from pancreatic alpha cells. In doing this, hepatic glucose is decreased and blood glucose is affected.[35] Because these medications act on the precursor to GLP-1 agonists, classwide A1c reduction is decreased when compared with GLP-1s (~0.8%). Additionally, it is important to discontinue DPP-4s when initiating a GLP-1 or visa versa as there is no additional benefit when taken together.[18]

Table 3
GLP-1 comparison table

Brand Name	Generic Name	Dosing Schedule	Additional Comments
Byetta	Exenatide	5–10 mcg subq twice daily	A1c reduction: 1% Weight loss: 2 kg Give an hour before breakfast and dinner, at least 6 h apart
Bydueron BCise	Exenatide ER	2 mg subq once weekly	A1c reduction: 1.5% Weight loss: 1.4–2.5 kg Available as an auto injector
Victoza	Liraglutide	0.6–1.8 mg subq once daily	A1c reduction: 1.5% Weight loss: 2.5 kg Need to prescribe pen needles Generic is FDA approved under brand name Saxenda for weight loss
Trulicity	Dulaglutide	0.75–1.5 mg subq once daily	A1c reduction: 1.5% Weight loss: 2.5 kg Needleless system for patients who do not want to "see" needle
Ozempic	Semaglutide	0.25-1 mg subq once weekly	A1c reduction: 1.5% Weight loss: 4 kg Pen needles supplied with pen FDA approved for weight loss under brand name Wegovy
Rybelsus	Semaglutide	7–14 mg by mouth once daily	A1c reduction: 1.4% Weight loss: 4.4 kg Only GLP-1 oral formulation Take 30 min before a meal with 4–6 oz of plain water

The proposed mechanism for cardiovascular benefit with DPP4s is that with increased glucose uptake comes increased ischemia tolerance as well as improvement in peripheral artery endothelial function.[36] However, in the CVOTs for the class, all agents were found to be noninferior to placebo when looking at MACE outcomes. In the SAVOR-TIMI53 and EXAMINE trial studying saxagliptin and alogliptin, respectively, there was an increased risk for hospitalization in patients with heart failure. While the risk was highest in patients with chronic kidney disease, preexisting heart failure, or elevated natriuretic peptides, the FDA added a warning label in 2016 to avoid saxagliptin and saxagliptin-containing products in heart failure patients.[37–39] The benefit of sitagliptin, linagliptin, saxagliptin, and alogliptin comes with their low level of adverse drug events. **Table 4** shows a comparison of the different medications within this medication class. These medications are typically used in needle adverse patients, not on a GLP-1 who need additional A1c reductions.[40]

Table 4
DPP4 comparison table

Brand Name	Generic Name	Dosing Schedule	Additional Comments
Januvia	Sitagliptin	Start & max: 100 mg daily CrCl 30–49: Max 50 mg daily CrCl <30: Max 25 mg daily	Combination product with metformin available
Onglyza	Saxagliptin	Start: 2.5–5 mg daily Max: 5 mg daily CrCl <50: Max 2.5 mg daily	Avoid in HF Combination product with metformin available CYP3A4 substrate; max dose 2.5 mg daily w/strong inhibitors
Tradjenta	Linagliptin	Start & Max: 5 mg daily	Only DPP4 with no renal dose adjustments Combination product available with metformin Combination product available with empagliflozin PGP & CYP3A4 substrate; do not use w/strong inhibitors
Nesina	Alogliptin	Start & Max: 25 mg once daily CrCl 30–60: 12.5 once daily CrCl 15–30: 6.25 once daily ESRD: 6.25 mg once daily	Avoid heart failure Combination product with metformin available Combination product with pioglitazone available

Sulfonylurea

Sulfonylureas are one of the oldest medications in the treatment of type 2 diabetes.[1] These medications, first discovered in 1946 and released to the public 10 years later, work to stimulate the beta cells in the pancreas, thus promoting insulin secretion.[41] They are still used as a cost-effective alternative that can lower A1c by as much as 1% to 2%. The sulfonylureas glipizide, glyburide, or glimepiride should be taken 30 minutes before eating a meal. With the high risk of hypoglycemia, caution should be used when pairing this medication with exogenous insulin agents, in patients who have missed meals, undernourished patients, patients abusing alcohol, and during hospitalizations.[42] One major counseling point for sulfonylureas is that due to the increased secretion of insulin, weight gain can be seen as a negative side effect. Additionally, sulfonylureas can lead to insulin burnout. Although there are conflicting theories as to whether this may be caused by hyperexcitation of B-cells or hypersecretion on insulin due to reduction in K_{ATP} channel activity, sulfonylureas have been shown to lead to pancreatic fatigue and reduction in blood glucose control within a few years of initiation.[43,44] As such, it is best practice to discontinue the medication after approximately 5 years of use.

As sulfonylureas were released to market before the 2008 CVOT requirements by the FDA, there is no large study looking into the effect of sulfonylureas on cardiovascular outcomes. However, there has been an increased risk of negative CV outcomes with patients using sulfonylureas as monotherapy. However, it is important to note that many of these trials were done as meta-analyses with different comparator drugs and varying degrees of design biases. Further studies are needed to identify true risk for increased CV and mortality outcomes.[45]

Table 5
Summary of Cardiovascular outcomes for the different medication classes

Class	Medication	CVOT Trial	Primary Outcome
DPP4	Saxagliptin[a]	SAVOR-TIMI 53	Nonsignificant 3 point MACE
	Alogliptin[a]	EXAMINE	Nonsignificant 3 point MACE
	Sitagliptin[b]	TECOS	Nonsignificant 4 point MACE
	Linagliptin[a]	CARMELINA	Nonsignificant 3 point MACE
GLP1	Lixisenatide[a]	ELIXA	Noninferior to placebo in 3 point MACE
	Liraglutide[a]	LEADER	Significant reduction in 3 point MACE
	Semaglutide SubQ[a]	SUSTAIN-6	Significant reduction in 3 point MACE
	Exenatide[a]	EXSCEL	Noninferior to placebo in 3 point MACE
	Dulaglutide[a]	REWIND	Significant reduction in 3 point MACE
	Semaglutide oral[a]	PIONEER-6	Noninferior to placebo in 3 point MACE
SGLT2	Empagliflozin[a]	EMPA-REG OUTCOME	Significant reduction in 3 point MACE
	Canagliflozin[a]	CANVAS	Significant reduction in 3 point MACE
	Dapagliflozin[a]	DECLARE-TIMI 58	Noninferior to placebo in 3 point MACE
	Ertugliflozin[a]	VERTIS-CV	Noninferior to placebo in 3 point MACE
	Dapagliflozin[a]	DAPA-HF	Significant reduction in the outcome of worsening HF or CV death in HFrEF
	Empagliflozin[a]	EMPA-REDUCED	Significant reduction in the outcome of worsening HF or CV death in HFrEF

[a] 3 point MACE: CV death, nonfatal MI, nonfatal stroke.
[b] 4 point MACE: CV death, nonfatal MI, nonfatal stroke, and hospitalization for unstable angina.

Thiazolidinediones

Thiazolidinediones (TZD) have fallen down the list of preferred options for treatment of type 2 diabetes, as they have not proven the same level of cardiovascular risk reduction as other classes. However, there is still a niche for them in therapy. This class increases insulin sensitization in peripheral tissues, including in the muscle, liver, and pancreas.[2] They are highly effective, reducing A1c by ~1.0%.[46] Pioglitazone has established benefit in nonalcoholic fatty liver disease, though the class has concerns in other disease states. Rosiglitazone was introduced to the market in 1999 and quickly gained popularity until data released in 2007 showed an increased risk of myocardial infarction.[47] The drug has been withdrawn in many countries, but is still available in the United States, though very rarely used. Pioglitazone use is associated with an increased risk of weight gain and edema, leading to an increased risk of heart failure exacerbations. There is also an increased risk of bone cancer in postmenopausal women and elderly men.[5] The 2021 ADA guidelines promote its use as an effective, low-cost option for patients who may have difficulty affording medications.[2]

DRUG CLASS REVIEW: PLACE IN THERAPY SUMMARY

In the treatment of T2DM, a wide variety of medications exist to help lower A1c and help reduce the risk of micro- and macro-vascular complications. It is important to use a patient-centered approach when selecting the appropriate agent. From analyzing side effect profiles and administration techniques to cost and other barriers to care, there are multiple variables to take into account when designing a treatment strategy to help a patient achieve their goals.

The most recent 2021 ADA guidelines strongly recommend initiation with metformin as first-line treatment, followed by dual therapy with either an SGLT2i or GLP-1 agent, particularly in patients who would benefit from weight loss, have ASCVD, or are at high risk for developing ASCVD, as both classes demonstrate significant A1c lowering, weight reduction, as well as cardiovascular and renal protection properties.[2] **Table 5** summarizes cardiovascular outcomes of the different medications in SGLT2i, GLP-1, and DPP4 drug classes. When deciding between the 2 classes of medication, the best practice advises counseling patients on the mechanism of action, expected side effects, administration of medication, and dosing—thus allowing the patient to participate in a shared decision-making process.

In patients who have established heart failure with reduced ejection fraction or established chronic kidney disease, SGLT2i agents are the preferred treatment after metformin initiation. **Table 6** demonstrates renal outcomes as studied in certain SGLT2i and GLP1 drug trials. In all of the above scenarios, if A1c is not at goal after dual therapy, it is recommended to escalate to triple therapy with metformin, an SGLT2i, and a GLP-1.

Table 6
Summary of renal outcomes for the different medication classes

Class	Medication	CVOT Trial	Outcome
GLP1	Liraglutide	LEADER Outcome studied: a composite of persistent macroalbuminuria, doubling of serum creatinine, ESRD, or death from ESRD	Significant reduction in the secondary outcome of new or worsening nephropathy
	Semaglutide SubQ	SUSTAIN-6 Outcome Studied: a composite of persistent UACR >300 mg/g Cr, doubling of serum creatinine, or ESRD	Significant reduction in the secondary outcome of new or worsening nephropathy
SGLT2	Empagliflozin	EMPA-REG OUTCOME Outcome Studied: a composite of progression to UACR >300 mg/g Cr, doubling of serum creatinine, ESRD, or death from ESRD	Significant reduction in the secondary outcome of incident or worsening nephropathy
	Canagliflozin	CREDENCE Outcome Studied: ESRD, doubling of serum creatinine, or renal or cardiovascular death	Significant reduction in the primary outcome
	Dapagliflozin	DAPA-CKD Outcome Studied: sustained decline in eGFR, end-stage kidney disease, or death from renal or cardiovascular causes	Significant reduction in the primary outcome

While concentrating on outcomes is important, the American Diabetes Association also recognizes the importance of addressing barriers to care. If a patient presents with cost concerns or is self-pay without access to medication assistance programs, agents such as thiazolidinediones and sulfonylureas can be used, albeit with lesser effect on A1c lowering and potentially greater risk for negative cardiovascular outcomes. In patients at high risk for hypoglycemia, using SGLT2i, GLP-1, DPP4, or TZDs is advised while avoiding sulfonylureas is advised. Significant advances in medication discovery and development have allowed clinicians to treat diabetes using a diverse arsenal of options. This wide array of medication classes allows for highly individualized therapy to improve diabetic control while keeping patient-centered care at the forefront of treatment goals.

CLINICS CARE POINTS

- Initiation of medication early on in the diagnosis of type 2 diabetes can limit negative outcomes and complications associated with uncontrolled diabetes

- Newer agents such as SGLT2i and GLP-1s have been fast-tracked to preferred classes of medications to be used in uncontrolled type 2 diabetes

- GLP-1s and SGLT2i seem to have class-wide safety in patients with ASCVD or heart failure, with most agents demonstrating cardiovascular risk reduction

- SGLT2i have demonstrated benefits in heart failure and renal disease. After metformin is initiated, SGLT2i is recommended for dual therapy.

- In the treatment of patients with type 2 diabetes, metformin remains the first line. Following a patient-centered treatment approach, GLP-1 or SGLT2i can be used in patients with ASCVD or ASCVD risk factors as well as in patients seeking additional weight loss benefits.

- Sulfonylureas and TZDs are reserved for patients with cost barriers or who are unable to tolerate an SGLT2i or a GLP-1.

- In patients who are at high risk for hypoglycemia, SGLT2i, GLP-1, TZD, or DPP4 can be used. Sulfonylureas should be avoided. Refer to other patient-specific factors listed above to determine the next steps in therapy.

DISCLOSURE

The authors have nothing to disclose. Neither author has commercial or financial conflicts of interest.

REFERENCES

1. White JR Jr. A brief history of the development of diabetes medications. Diabetes Spectr 2014;27(2):82–6.
2. American Diabetes Association. 9. Pharmacologic approaches to glycemic treatment: standards of medical care in diabetes-2021. Diabetes Care 2021; 44(Supplement 1):S111–24.
3. Holman RR, Paul SK, Bethel MA, et al. 10-year follow-up of intensive glucose control in type 2 diabetes. N Engl J Med 2008;359:1577–89.
4. Bailey CJ, Turner RC. Metformin. N Engl J Med 1996;334(9):574–9.
5. Garber AJ, Handelsman Y, Grunberger G, et al. Diabetes management algorithm. Endocr Pract 2020;26(1):107–39.

6. Reinstatler L, Qi YP, Williamson RS, et al. Association of biochemical B12 deficiency with metformin therapy and vitamin B12 supplements. Diabetes Care 2012;35:327–33.

7. American Diabetes Association. 3. Prevention or delay of type 2 diabetes: standards of medical care in diabetes-2021. Diabetes Care 2021;44(Supplement 1): S34–9. https://doi.org/10.2337/dc21-S003.

8. Johnson NP. Metformin use in women with polycystic ovary syndrome. Ann Transl Med 2014;2(6):56. https://doi.org/10.3978/j.issn.2305-5839.2014.04.15.

9. Hsia DS, Grove D, Cefalu WT. An update on SGLT inhibitors for the treatment of diabetes mellitus. Curr Opin Endocrinol Diabetes Obes 2017;24(1):73–9.

10. FDA. FDA revises labels of SGLT2 inhibitors for diabetes to include warnings about too much acid in the blood and serious urinary tract infections. 2020. Available at: https://www.fda.gov/drugs/drug-safety-and-availability/fda-revises-labels-sglt2-inhibitors-diabetes-include-warnings-about-too-much-acid-blood-and-serious. Accessed July 8, 2021.

11. US. Food and Drug Administration. Guidance for industry: diabetes mellitus 2008. Available at: www.fda.gov/downloads/Drugs/GuidanceComplianceRegulatory Information/Guidances/ucm071627.pdf. Accessed July 8, 2021.

12. Zinman B, Wanner C, Lachin JM, et al. Empagliflozin, cardiovascular outcomes, and mortality in type 2 diabetes. N Engl J Med 2015;373:2117–28.

13. Neal B, Perkovic B, Mahaffey KW, et al. Canagliflozin and cardiovascular and renal events in type 2 diabetes. N Engl J Med 2017;377:644–57.

14. McMurray JV, Solomon SD, Inzucchi SE. Dapagliflozin in patients with heart failure and reduced ejection fraction. N Engl J Med 2019;381:1995–2008.

15. Packer M, Anker S, Butler J, et al. Cardiovascular and renal outcomes with empagliflozin in heart failure. N Engl J Med 2020;383:1413–24.

16. Farxiga. Package insert. Astra Zeneca Pharmaceuticals LP; 2020.

17. Perkovic V, Jardine MJ, Neal B, et al. Canagliflozin and renal outcomes in type 2 diabetes and nephropathy. N Engl J Med 2019;380:2295–306.

18. Heerspink HJL, Stefansson BV, Correa-Rotter R, et al. Dapagliflozin in patients with chronic kidney disease. N Engl J Med 2020;383:1436–46.

19. Drucker DJ, Nauck MA. The incretin system: glucagon-like peptide-1 receptor agonists and dipeptidyl peptidase-4 inhibitors in type 2 diabetes. Lancet 2006; 368:1696–705. https://doi.org/10.1016/S0140-6736(06)69705-5.

20. Shah M, Vella A. Effects of GLP-1 on appetite and weight. Rev Endocr Metab Disord 2014;15(3):181–7. https://doi.org/10.1007/s11154-014-9289-5.

21. Saxenda. Package insert. Novo Nordisk; 2020.

22. Wegovy. Package insert. Novo Nordisk; 2021.

23. Filippatos TD, Panagiotopoulou TV, Elisaf MS. Adverse Effects of GLP-1 Receptor Agonists. Rev Diabetic Stud 2014;11(3–4):202–30. https://doi.org/10.1900/RDS. 2014.11.202.

24. Dietle A, Campanale M, Ostroff S. GLP-1 receptor agonists: an alternative for rapid-acting insulin? US Pharm 2016;41(10):3–6.

25. Pratley R, Amod A, Hoff ST, et al. Oral semaglutide versus subcutaneous liraglutide and placebo in type 2 diabetes (PIONEER 4): a randomised, double-blind, phase 3a trial. Lancet 2019;394:39–50.

26. Sheahan K, Wahlerg E, Gilbert M. An overview of GLP-1 agonists and recent cardiovascular outcomes trials. Postgrad Med J 2019;0:1–6. https://doi.org/10.1136/postgradmedj-2019-137186.

27. Pfeffer MA, Claggett B, Diaz R, et al. Lixisenatide in patients with type 2 diabetes and acute coronary syndrome. N Engl J Med 2015;373:2247–57.

28. Marso SP, Daniels GH, Brown-Frandsen K, et al. Liraglutide and cardiovascular outcomes in type 2 diabetes. N Engl J Med 2016;375:311–22.

29. Marso SP, Bain SC, Consoli A, et al. Semaglutide and cardiovascular outcomes in patients with type 2 diabetes. N Engl J Med 2016;375:1834–44.

30. Holman RR, Bethel MA, Mentz RJ, et al. Effects of once-weekly exenatide on cardiovascular outcomes in type 2 diabetes. N Engl J Med 2017;377:1228–39.

31. Hernandez AF, Green JB, Janmohamed S, et al. Albiglutide and cardiovascular outcomes in patients with type 2 diabetes and cardiovascular disease (HARMONY OUTCOMES): a double-blind, randomised placebo-controlled trial. Lancet 2018;392:1519–29.

32. Gerstein HC, Colhoun HM, Dagenais GR, et al. Dulaglutide and cardiovascular outcomes in type 2 diabetes (REWIND): a double-blind, randomised placebo controlled trial. Lancet 2019;394:121–30.

33. Husain M, Birkenfeld AL, Donsmark M, et al. Oral Semaglutide and cardiovascular outcomes in patients with type 2 diabetes. N Engl J Med 2019;381:841–51.

34. Yin WL, Bain SC, Min T. The effect of glucagon-like peptide-1 receptor agonists on renal outcomes in type 2 diabetes. Diabetes Ther 2020;11(4):835–44. https://doi.org/10.1007/s13300-020-00798-x.

35. Gallwitz B. Clinical use of DPP-4 inhibitors. Front Endocrinol 2019;10:389. https://doi.org/10.3389/fendo.2019.00389.

36. Zhang Z, Chen X, Lu P, et al. Incretin-based agents in type 2 diabetic patients at cardiovascular risk: compare the effect of GLP-1 agonists and DPP-4 inhibitors on cardiovascular and pancreatic outcomes. Cardiovasc Diabetol 2017;16:31.

37. Scirica BM, Bhatt DL, Braunwald E, et al. Saxagliptin and cardiovascular outcomes in patients with type 2 diabetes mellitus. N Engl J Med 2013;369(14):1317–26. https://doi.org/10.1056/NEJMoa1307684.

38. White W, Cannon C, Heller S, et al. Alogliptin after acute coronary syndrome in patients with type 2 diabetes. N Engl J Med 2013;369:1327–37. https://doi.org/10.1056/NEJMoa1305889.

39. Center for Drug Evaluation and Research. FDA drug safety communication: FDA adds warnings about heart failure risk to labels of type 2 diabetes medicines containing saxagliptin and alogliptin. U.S. Food and Drug Administration. Available at: https://www.fda.gov/drugs/drug-safety-and-availability/fda-drug-safety-communication-fda-adds-warnings-about-heart-failure-risk-labels-type-2-diabetes. Accessed July 8, 2021.

40. Nauck MA, Meier JJ, Cavender MA, et al. Cardiovascular actions and clinical outcomes with glucagon-like peptide-1 receptor agonists and dipeptidyl peptidase-4 inhibitors. Circulation 2017;136(9):849–70. https://doi.org/10.1161/CIRCULATIONAHA.117.028136.

41. Levine R. Sulfonylureas: Background and development of the field. Diabetes Care 1984;7(Suppl 1):3–7.

42. Gangji AS, Cukierman T, Gerstein HC, et al. A systematic review and meta-analysis of hypoglycemia and cardiovascular events: a comparison of glyburide with other secretagogues and with insulin. Diabetes Care 2007;30:389–94.

43. Matthews DR, Cull CA, Stratton IM, et al. UKPDS 26: Sulphonylurea failure in non-insulin-dependent diabetic patients over six years. UK Prospective Diabetes Study (UKPDS) Group. Diabet Med 1998;15:297–303.

44. Donath M, Ehses J, Maedler K, et al. Mechanisms of B-cell death in type 2 diabetes. Diabetes 2005;54(suppl 2):S108–13. https://doi.org/10.2337/diabetes.54.suppl_2.S108.

45. Azoulay L, Suissa S. Sulfonylureas and the risks of cardiovascular events and death: a methodological meta-regression analysis of the observational studies. Diabetes Care 2017;40(5):706–14. https://doi.org/10.2337/dc16-1943.

46. Wang W, Zhou X, Kwong JSW, et al. Efficacy and safety of thiazolidinediones in diabetes patients with renal impairment: a systematic review and meta-analysis. Sci Rep 2017;7:1717. https://doi.org/10.1038/s41598-017-01965-0.

47. Center for Drug Evaluation and Research. FDA requires removal of some prescribing and dispensing restriction. U.S. Food and Drug Administration. Available at: https://www.fda.gov/drugs/drug-safety-and-availability/fda-drug-safety-communication-fda-requires-removal-some-prescribing-and-dispensing-restrictions. Accessed July 8, 2021.

Diabetes and Technology

Kelsey Simmons, DO[a], Sterling Riddley, MD[b],*

KEYWORDS

- Continuous glucose monitoring • Insulin pump • Hybrid closed loop
- Smart insulin pen

KEY POINTS

- Three available means to assess glycemic values are hemoglobin A_{1c}, self-monitoring of blood glucose (SMBG), and continuous glucose monitoring (CGM), each with its own strengths and limitations.
- Mobile applications are making it easier for glycemic data to be consolidated into actionable reports, guiding treatment decisions, and making long-acting insulin titration easier for patients.
- Continuous glucose monitoring is an emerging technology used to improve patient outcomes and public health.
- CGM software is making it easier for clinicians and patients to share glycemic data to achieve greater glycemic control in less time.
- Insulin pump therapy is a safe and effective treatment of patients with type 1 or type 2 diabetes.
- Continuous glucose monitors can work with insulin pumps to provide sensor-augmented and automated delivery of insulin.

INTRODUCTION

Three available means to assess glycemic control are (1) hemoglobin A_{1c}, (HbA_{1c}), (2) self-monitoring of blood glucose (SMBG), and (3) continuous glucose monitoring (CGM).[1] HbA_{1c}, the gold standard for monitoring glycemic control and predicting complications, has certain limitations: it does not distinguish among fasting, preprandial, and postprandial hyperglycemia; it fails to recognize glycemic excursions or variability; it does not identify resolution of hypoglycemia; and it does not provide immediate feedback to patients about lifestyle factors that influence glycemic control.[2]

SMBG can resolve the limitations in the use of HbA_{1c}.[2] SMBG can guide management strategies, improve problem-solving skills, and shorten the time interval in which patients achieve a goal HbA_{1c}, as demonstrated in type 1 diabetes, insulin-treated and

[a] Family Medicine, UNC Health Southeastern Gray's Creek Medical Clinic, 1249 Chicken Foot Road, Hope Mills, NC 28348, USA; [b] Duke/Southern Regional Area Health Education Center, 1601 Owen Drive, Fayetteville, NC 28304, USA
* Corresponding author.
E-mail address: sterling.riddley@sr-ahec.org

Prim Care Clin Office Pract 49 (2022) 327–337
https://doi.org/10.1016/j.pop.2021.11.005
0095-4543/22/© 2021 Elsevier Inc. All rights reserved.

primarycare.theclinics.com

non-insulin-treated type 2 diabetes, pregnant patients with diabetes, and children with diabetes.[2,3] However, SMBG also has limitations: data achieved by SMBG represent single points in time and fail to assess glycemic variability, frequency of testing, accuracy of reporting, difficulty in obtaining overnight data, and missed hypoglycemic episodes.[1]

CGM, an emerging technology that helps fill the gaps in glycemic monitoring found with HbA$_{1c}$ and SMBG, provides instantaneous, real-time display of glucose level and rate of change of glucose, alerts patients for actual or impending hypoglycemia and hyperglycemia, provides daytime and overnight coverage, and assesses glycemic variability.[4] Additional benefits of CGM include reductions in HbA$_{1c}$ and glycemic variability, increased time in target glycemic range, decreased time in hypoglycemic range, and fewer hypoglycemic events.[5] Use of CGM is expected to increase with concomitant increases in patient outcomes and public health.[4] Here we review some of the available tools that facilitate the advancement of CGM use.

MOBILE APPLICATIONS FOR MONITORING OF BLOOD GLUCOSE AND INSULIN TITRATION

For clinicians managing patients with diabetes on multiple daily injections of insulin, the volume of data generated through SMBG is often difficult to interpret. For patients, the titration of insulin is confusing. Mobile applications are emerging to overcome these difficulties. Glooko's (Mountain View, CA) Mobile Insulin Dosing System (MIDS) and Voluntis' (Cambridge, MA) Insulia app are making it easier and less intimidating for patients to self-titrate basal insulin therapy.

Glooko, an online platform used for in-clinic and remote diabetes management, uses data contained in standard glucometers to consolidate blood glucose readings into actionable insights enabling treatment decisions.[6] Data from a glucometer are synced onto either a mobile application on a patient's smart device or through a USB connection between the glucometer and a Glooko transmitter for in-office use.[6] That information is then used to generate reports containing pertinent information, such as average blood glucose, in-range blood glucose, and trends of recurrent hyperglycemia and hypoglycemia for use in clinical practice.[6] Glooko is compatible with 95% of all glucometers.[6]

MIDS and Insulia mobile application (or web portal system) are interactive applications that assist in titrating long-acting insulin doses.[7,8] Both applications allow a clinician to generate a treatment plan that provides guidance on long-acting insulin dosing.[7,8] Insulia is offered as a prescription-only application.[8] The treatment plan is conveyed to the patient via the Glooko Mobile Application on the patient's smart device or via emailed login credentials for the Insulia app.[7,8] The MIDS reminds the patient to check their blood glucose, computes how much insulin the patient should take, and reminds the patient to take their insulin.[7] On the Insulia app, the patient enters blood glucose values into the app, which provides real-time insulin dose recommendations as outlined in the treatment plan.[8] The clinician can remotely monitor progress via the Insulia web portal, making adjustments if needed.[8] These applications simplify insulin dosing and prevent poor outcomes for people taking insulin.[7,8]

PERSONAL CONTINUOUS GLUCOSE MONITORING

Personal CGM systems are available for at-home, daily monitoring of blood glucose. Patient populations eligible for personal CGM systems include patients with type 1 or type 2 diabetes on intensive insulin therapy and not meeting glucose targets or who are experiencing hypoglycemic episodes.[9] The patient uses a receiver, smartphone, smartwatch, or another compatible device to receive continuously transmitted glucose data.[9] Additional features include alerts and alarms for rising or falling glucose levels and the ability to share data remotely with family, caregivers, and clinicians.[9] There are currently four available personal CGM devices: FreeStyle Libre (Abbott, Alameda, CA), Dexcom G6 (Dexcom, San Diego, CA), Medtronic Guardian Sensor 3 (Minneapolis, MN), and Eversense (Eversense, Germantown, MD).[9]

The FreeStyle Libre 14-day and FreeStyle Libre 2 are two available intermittently scanned CGM systems that require users to scan their sensors to obtain blood glucose data.[9,10] The FreeStyle Libre 14-day system does not have alarms, whereas the FreeStyle Libre 2 has optional alarms.[9,10] Each device uses trend arrows to inform the patient if sensor glucose is stable, rising, or falling.[9,10] The FreeStyle Libre 14-day and the Freestyle Libre 2 are used with a separate receiver or smartphone.[9,10] This system does not require fingerstick blood glucose calibration to ensure the accuracy of glucose readings and cannot be integrated with an insulin pump.[9,10]

The Dexcom G6 CGM, a real-time CGM device that does not require fingerstick blood glucose calibration, comes with its own receiver.[9] Additionally, other platforms (Android and Apple smartphones, smartwatches, and Tandem t:slim X2 insulin pump [San Diego, CA]) are used to obtain glycemic data.[9] Data are remotely shared with family, caregivers, and clinicians.[9] The sensor is worn for up to 10 days and alerts are activated when a glucose value less than or equal to 55 mg/dL is predicted within the next 20 minutes.[9,11]

The Medtronic Guardian Sensor 3 is a real-time CGM device that requires finger-stick blood glucose calibration at least twice daily to ensure accuracy of glucose readings.[9] Compatible receivers include the Guardian Connect application on Apple devices.[9] Data are remotely shared with family, caregivers, and clinicians.[9] This device is compatible with the Minmed 630G and 670G insulin pumps.[9] The sensor is worn for 7 days.[9]

Eversense is a CGM device consisting of a 90-day implantable CGM sensor with an external transmitter worn over the sensor.[12,13] The rechargeable, battery-powered transmitter (which is removed without the need for sensor replacement) wirelessly initiates the transfer of data to the sensor every 5 minutes through a secured low-energy Bluetooth transmission to a mobile medical application.[13] Hypoglycemic and hyperglycemic alerts are provided on a mobile device in addition to on-body vibratory alerts if a mobile device is not nearby.[13] This device was designed to reduce the inconvenience and discomfort of weekly sensor insertions and improve lifestyle flexibility.[13] Important contraindications to the use of this system include the concomitant use of immunosuppressant therapy, chemotherapy, systemic glucocorticoids, or anticoagulant therapy; those with another active implantable device; and those with known allergies to systemic glucocorticoids.[9]

PROFESSIONAL CONTINUOUS GLUCOSE MONITORING

Some challenges involved with personal CGM use include insurance coverage limitations and patient preference.[12] A professional CGM system is a reasonable alternative to personal CGM and does not require the patient to purchase their own system.[12] A professional CGM is purchased by a clinic and used intermittently by patients as prescribed.[9] The equipment is returned to the clinic after use where data are downloaded and analyzed to improve clinical decisions.[9] The current standard of care for reproducible pattern recognition is to analyze 14 days of CGM data.[12] The data can then be reviewed with the patient to improve clinical decision-making strategies or inform self-management skills.[9,12] One pertinent distinction between the use of a personal or a professional CGM is the professional systems' ability to blind glycemic data.[9] Blinded data are used to further explain the indications for starting insulin therapy, gives patients a clear image of a specific problem, and arguably represents patients' typical lifestyle factors that determine glycemic levels throughout the study period.[9] Currently, three systems are marketed for professional CGM use in the United States: Medtronic iPro2 system, Dexcom G6 Pro, and FreeStyle Libre Pro.[12]

The Medtronic iPro2 is a blinded system consisting of a sensor with an attached data storage component, approved for patients aged 16 years and older.[9,12] The Medtronic Enlite sensor is worn for 7 days at a time and is reused by multiple patients with proper disinfection.[9] The patient is required to perform SMBG four times per day during the trial period and bring a log of these readings to the interpretation visit.[9] SMBG readings are then entered into CareLink iPro therapy management software, which generates a report for analysis.[9]

The Dexcom G6 Pro is approved for ages 2 years and older. The system includes a sensor, transmitter, and reader.[12] Sensors are worn for 10 days, and the transmitter and the sensor are for single use only. The reader is used to verify sensor start because it does not display CGM data.[9] No SMBG calibration is required. The Dexcom G6 Pro is blinded or unblinded; those who wish to be unblinded to sensor sugars need to have a smartphone compatible with the Dexcom G6 app. After 10 days, data are extracted using the reader and uploaded to Dexcom Clarity.

The FreeStyle Libre Pro CGM, approved for ages 18 and older, consists of a factory-calibrated, 14-day sensor applied to the back of the upper arm.[10,12] Glucose levels are measured every minute and the sensor stores data automatically every 15 minutes.[10] The stored data are then retrieved using either a dedicated reader device or smartphone.[10] Available information includes the current glucose level, a trend arrow showing the direction of glucose excursion, and a graph of glucose readings over the preceding 8 hours.[10] On completion of the 14-day trial period, the sensor is discarded and cannot be reused.[9] The FreeStyle LibreView software is used to download the stored data to be analyzed by the clinician.[9]

CONTINUOUS GLUCOSE MONITORING SOFTWARE

Glycemic data received by transmitters are shared remotely with family, caregivers, and clinicians, and various software is used to download stored data for analysis by clinicians. Each CGM platform uses its own unique software: the Dexcom CLARITY diabetes management application, the FreeStyle LibreLink and LibreLinkUp app, the Medtronic CareLink reports, and the Eversense Data Management System.[14–17]

The Dexcom CLARITY app is downloaded to a compatible smart device and has two user functionalities: Dexcom CLARITY for home users (to be used by the patient) and Dexcom CLARITY for clinics (to be used by the health care professional).[14] The patient connects the Dexcom receiver to upload and view glucose data as graphs, trends, statistics, and day-by-day readings.[14] This information can then be printed for or emailed to the health care provider from the Dexcom CLARITY World Wide Web page.[14] The patient can also generate a sharing code, which can be given to the clinician[14] and then entered into the Dexcom Web site by the health care professional for analysis and interpretation.[14]

FreeStyle Libre has two platforms that allow patients and clinicians to view saved data: the LibreLink, which the patient uses to monitor their glucose; and the LibreLinkUp, used by family members or clinicians to view the saved glucose information.[15] LibreLink is downloaded onto a compatible smart device and provides the patient with the current glucose reading, trend arrows, and glucose history for the last 8 hours.[15]

The patient can also add notations, such as food intake, insulin use, or exercise.[15] Data are stored for up to 90 days.[15] LibreLinkUp, which is downloaded to a compatible smart device, allows up to 20 people to remotely track the patient's glucose data and trends through the use of a share invitation provided by the patient.[15]

Medtronic CareLink is a free, World Wide Web–based program that collects information from Medtronic CGM devices to generate reports and monitor progress.[16] The patient creates an account on the CareLink Personal homepage and uses an uploader application to upload data from the CGM device.[16] From there, the patient can generate reports to be shared with the provider.[16]

The Eversense Data Management System is a World Wide Web–based platform in which the patient and the clinician register separate accounts.[17,18] Those two accounts are then linked, either by the provider sending the patient an invitation or the patient requesting to join a particular clinic.[18] Once the two accounts are linked, the patient and clinician can view various glucose statistics and generate reports to assist in clinical decision-making.[18]

INSULIN PUMP THERAPY

Continuous subcutaneous insulin infusion, or insulin pump therapy, has had significant technological advancements over the years. Insulin pumps are programmable devices that administer short- or rapid-acting insulin in a basal and bolus fashion to mimic a patient's physiologic insulin demands.[19] Insulin pumps are divided into two groups: tubed and tubeless. Tubed insulin pumps have several components: subcutaneous cannula, infusion set, delivery line tubing, insulin reservoir, display, and operating buttons that may or may not be a touch screen (**Table 1**).[20] Tubed insulin pumps use infusion sets, which consist of tubing that carries insulin from the pump to the patient; as one end attaches to the reservoir, the other end attaches to the insertion site on the patient. The reservoir holds the insulin and can vary in size from 200 to 300 units of rapid-acting insulin. Tubeless insulin pumps attach directly to the skin and are controlled with a handheld device known as a personal diabetes manager (PDM).

Patients that are on continuous subcutaneous insulin infusion no longer require long-acting insulin to control fasting blood sugar. Basal insulin is a constant infusion

Table 1 Insulin pump components	
Insulin Pump Component	**Definition and Function**
Reservoir	Insulin supply
Cannula	Tube inserted into tissue subcutaneously in which insulin is delivered to the body
Tubing	Brings insulin from the pump to the infusion set
Infusion set	Connects the insulin pump delivery device to the patient's body (cannula + tubing)
Insulin pump	Device that houses the insulin reservoir and stores insulin pump settings (tubed pumps)
Personal diabetes manager	Handheld device used to wirelessly manage insulin delivery and house insulin pump settings in tubeless insulin pump (Omnipod)

Data from Paldus B, Lee MH, O'Neal DN. Insulin pumps in general practice. Aust Prescr. 2018 Dec;41(6):186-190.

of rapid-acting insulin measured in units per hour. Insulin pumps allow for multiple programmable basal rates throughout the day, factoring in a patient's physical activity, work schedule, exercise, illness, and individual physiology.[21] Patients with type 1 or type 2 diabetes that is not well-controlled on multiple daily injections may see improved glycemic control with fewer episodes of hypoglycemia when transitioned to continuous subcutaneous insulin infusion.[22–24]

Boluses are doses of rapid-acting insulin that cover food/carbohydrates or bring down elevated glucose readings (correction bolus). The bolus calculator is a program integrated into insulin pump software that allows patients to dose insulin for carbohydrates and high blood sugars. A bolus calculator can help patients meet prandial insulin dosage requirements more accurately and improve postprandial glycemic excursions.[25] The bolus calculator uses the insulin-to- carbohydrate ratio (I:C), sensitivity factor, glucose target, insulin duration, and insulin on board to ensure patients receive the correct amount of insulin.

The I:C is the number of grams of carbohydrates that one unit of insulin will cover. Accurate carbohydrate counting and use of the I:C have been shown to lower HbA_{1c} more than giving a fixed or estimated bolus to cover meals.[26] Carbohydrate boluses are given for carbohydrates consumed during meals or snacks not intended to raise or prevent low blood sugar. Meals with different fat and protein content can affect a patient's blood sugar; high-fat/high-protein meals can cause more frequent postprandial hyperglycemia than foods of identical carbohydrate content but lower-fat/lower-protein content.[27,28] Extended bolus features allow patients to administer a bolus over a selected period, often used when eating a long meal with extended snacking, history gastroparesis, or high-fat/high-protein meals.[29,30] Insulin pumps allow for predetermined/fixed doses of mealtime insulin for patients that are not proficient at carbohydrate counting. A correction bolus is administered if blood sugars are greater than the desired target. This dose is determined by the target blood sugar, insulin sensitivity, and insulin on board using a bolus calculator (**Table 2**).[20]

Table 2
Insulin pump terminology

Terminology	Definition
Basal rate	The rate at which an insulin pump provides small, "background" doses of fast-acting insulin, used to maintain glucose during fasting states
Bolus dose	The "on-demand" delivery of rapid-acting insulin for food and blood glucose
Insulin-to-carbohydrate ratio	The number of grams of carbohydrates that one unit of insulin will cover
Insulin sensitivity/correction factor	The amount in mg/dL a patient's blood sugar will drop with one unit insulin
Insulin action time (insulin duration)	How long insulin takes to finish lowering glucose
Insulin on board	Insulin that is still active in one's body from previous bolus doses
Target glucose	Desired glucose level
Total daily dose of insulin	Total amount of insulin a patient requires in a 24-h period (basal + bolus)

Data from Paldus B, Lee MH, O'Neal DN. Insulin pumps in general practice. Aust Prescr. 2018 Dec;41(6):186-190.

Sensor-Augmented and Automated Insulin Delivery/Hybrid Closed Loop Devices

Continuous glucose monitors can work with insulin pumps to deliver insulin through nonautomated delivery (sensor-augmented) and automated delivery (hybrid closed-loop). Sensor augmented pumps allow patients to see their glucose levels on their insulin pumps or a separate device, alerting them if their glucose levels rise or fall.[31] In addition, a sensor-augmented pump can allow for the automatic suspension of basal insulin if sensor glucose is below or is approaching a predetermined low glucose limit, with the ability to restart the basal insulin once the sensor glucose has reached an appropriate level.[31,32] Sensor-augmented pump therapy effectively lowers blood sugar without increasing the risk for hypoglycemia compared with patients treated with multiple daily injections.[33]

In a hybrid closed-loop system, the insulin pump works in conjunction with a continuous glucose monitor and algorithm to deliver rapid-acting insulin automatically.[32] The algorithm allows for basal insulin to be increased, decreased, stopped, and resumed depending on the current and predicted sensor glucose. Some hybrid closed-loop systems also administer a correction bolus for elevated sensor sugar. Current hybrid closed-loop systems cannot administer automatic mealtime insulin doses. Patients should be encouraged to bolus before meals to prevent postmeal hyperglycemia, unnecessary automated basal adjustment, or administration of automatic correction bolus.[32]

Available Insulin Pumps

Insulet's (Acton, MA) Omnipod and Omnipod Dash insulin pump systems are tubeless pumps composed of disposable pods and a PDM. The disposable pods require no tubing or infusion sets and are placed directly on the skin for up to 72 hours while holding up to 200 units of U-100 insulin.[34] Insulin pump settings are programmed into the PDM, which communicate wirelessly through bidirectional radio frequency communication with the Omnipod and Bluetooth technology with the Omnipod Dash.[34] Both systems adjust basal rates in increments of 0.05 units per hour with a maximum basal rate of 30 units per hour and deliver boluses in increments of 0.05 units with a maximum of 30 units.[34] In addition, the Omnipod Dash allows for the basal rate to be set at 0 units per hour. Neither the Omnipod nor the Omnipod Dash is currently compatible with a CGM.[32] Insulet's Omnipod 5 system is seeking Food and Drug Administration approval as a tubeless hybrid closed-loop insulin pump, compatible with Dexcom G6; early studies have shown that it is safe and effective for adults and children with type 1 diabetes.[35]

Medtronic Minimed currently offers three different insulin pumps in the United States (Medtronic 630G, 670G, and 770G), all with SmartGuard technology. SmartGuard technology automatically adjusts basal insulin delivery by suspending or resuming basal insulin based on a patient's sensor glucose values and low limits. The Medtronic 630G with SmartGuard technology is a sensor-augmented pump that works in conjunction with the Guardian 3 CGM. Medtronic's hybrid closed-loop system insulin pumps, the 670G and 770G, allow for sensor-augmented and automatic insulin delivery when used with the Guardian 3 CGM.[36,37] The 670G and 770G pumps differ only in that the latter has Bluetooth capability; both systems use the same algorithm for its automated insulin delivery. Each pump can work in two modes: manual mode and auto mode. In manual mode, the system functions as a sensor-augmented pump when used with Guardian CGM.[38,39] In auto mode, the pump works as a hybrid closed-loop system to maintain a target sensor sugar of 120 mg/dL, with the option to increase target glucose to 150 mg/dL during heavy activity to avoid hypoglycemia.[32] Clinician preprogrammed I:C are used for administering insulin for meals while in auto mode.[37] Correction bolus is operational while in auto mode with a target of 150 mg/dL using the insulin sensitivity/correction factor and I:C settings programmed by the clinician.[32] Medtronic's hybrid closed-loop system has shown the ability to lower time in range, decrease HbA$_{1c}$, and reduce hypoglycemia in patients with type 1 diabetes.[40]

Tandem's t:slim X2 is a tubed insulin pump that is touch screen controlled and holds up to 300 units of U-100 insulin.[41] The t:slim X2 adjusts basal rates in increments of 0.001 units per hour with a maximum basal rate of 15 units per hour and delivers boluses in increments of 0.01 units with a maximum of 25 units.[41] The t:slim X2 is compatible with the Dexcom G6, allowing patients to visualize their sensor readings on their pump screen.[32] Tandem's t:slim X2 insulin pump offers remote software updates and data sharing via the t:connect mobile app.[42] It also offers patients two CGM-assisted insulin delivery options: Basal-IQ:suspend before low (sensor-augmented insulin delivery) and Control-IQ (a closed hybrid loop system), both with the Dexcom G6 CGM. Basal-IQ technology uses Dexcom G6 CGM values to predict glucose levels 30 minutes ahead; if glucose levels are expected to be less than 80 mg/dL or if a reading falls to less than 70 mg/dL, insulin delivery suspends.[43] Insulin delivery resumes as soon as sensor glucose values begin to rise, which may be for a minimum of 5 minutes and a maximum of 2 hours.[43] The use of Basal-IQ technology can reduce episodes of hypoglycemia.[44] Control-IQ technology can adjust insulin delivery by increasing, decreasing, or suspending basal insulin when sensor glucose values are predicted to be less than 112.5 mg/dL or greater than 160 mg/dL.[41] The system delivers an automatic correction bolus at 60% of the calculated dose with a target of 110 mg/dL, no more than once an hour if sensor glucose is predicted to be greater than 180 mg/dL.[32,41] Tandem's t:slim X2 Control-IQ technology can result in more time in range, less time with hypoglycemia, and better HbA$_{1c}$ than patients on an insulin pump and CGM therapy not using Control-IQ.[45]

SMART INSULIN PEN

Insulins pumps are not the only technology that allows patients to use a bolus calculator to help dose mealtime insulin. The InPen (Medtronic) is a home-use reusable manual pen injector containing a nonreplaceable battery and electronics that communicate via Bluetooth with the InPen app on Apple or Android devices.[46] The InPen battery lasts a year without the need for charging. In addition, the pen injector is compatible with 3-mL cartridges of U-100 insulin along with single-use detachable and disposable needles.[46] The pen injector allows the user to dial the desired dose from 0.5 to 30 units in 0.5-unit increments.[46]

The app comes equipped with a bolus dose calculator for which the clinician enters the settings (consisting of the I:C, insulin sensitivity/correction factor, glucose target range, insulin duration, and maximum calculated dose).[47] The dose calculator recommends the amount of insulin needed to keep the blood sugar in the target range while factoring present blood sugar, estimated carbohydrate intake, and insulin on board while recording the amount of insulin the patient administers.[47] The app allows the clinician to set up fixed or variable meal sizes for patients who are not proficient at carb counting.[47] Along with dosing insulin, the InPen app also allows for data integration from a patient's CGM; currently, the InPen is compatible with the Dexcom G6 CGM and Medtronic Guardian Connect system.[46] This integration allows for reports to be printed and reviewed by the clinician, detailing the dose of insulin given and the patient's response to the dose.[47]

SUMMARY

Diabetes technology is designed to improve the health of people with diabetes, using CGM, mobile applications with insulin dosing titration, cloud-based data sharing, Bluetooth-enabled insulin pens, and insulin pump therapy. The use of CGM provides helpful information to the patient and clinician that is not evident with SMBG and HbA$_{1c}$. Sensor augmented and hybrid closed-loop systems allow for integrating CGM technology in insulin pumps to treat patients with diabetes effectively and safely.

CLINICS CARE POINTS

- Diabetes technology can benefit patients of all ages.
- Patients who are at increased risk for hypoglycemia may have a more significant benefit with a CGM that has hypoglycemia alarms.
- Insulin pump and CGM compatibility should be considered when selecting insulin pumps and CGMs.
- Insulin pump therapy is a safe and effective treatment of patients with type 1 or type 2 diabetes requiring multiple doses of insulin.
- Patients on hybrid closed-loop systems should continue to bolus for carbohydrates.

CONFLICT OF INTEREST

The authors have no commercial or financial conflicts of interest.

REFERENCES

1. Wright E, Gavin J. Clinical use of professional continuous glucose monitoring. Diabetes Technology Ther 2017;19(2):S12–5.
2. Parkin C, Davidson J. Value of self-monitoring blood glucose pattern analysis in improving diabetes outcome. J Diabetes Sci Technology 2009;3(3):500–8.
3. Miller KM, Beck RW, Bergenstal RM, et al. Evidence of a strong association between frequency of self-monitoring of blood glucose and hemoglobin a1c levels in t1d exchange clinic registry participants. Diabetes Care 2013;36:2009–13.
4. Rodbard D. Continuous glucose monitoring: a review of successes, challenges, and opportunities. Diabetes Technology Ther 2016;18:13, 2 S2-3 to S2.
5. Anderson J, Gavin J, Kruger DF, et al. Current eligibility requirements for CGM coverage are harmful, costly, and unjustified. Diabetes Technology Ther 2020; 22(3):169–73.
6. Glooko simplify collaboration. 2021. Available at: https://www.glooo.com/. June 28, 2021.
7. Beadle R. Glooko's mobile insulin dosing system – MIDS – is FDA cleared. 2018. Available at: https://www.glooko.com/2018/02/glookos-mobile-insulin-dosing-system-mids-fda-cleared/. June 28, 2021.
8. Voluntis. Insulia: Helping you get to the right dose. Every Day. 2017-2020. Available at: https://insulia.com/. June 28, 2021.
9. Longo R, Sperling S. Personal versus professional continuous glucose monitoring: when to use which on whom. From Res Pract 2019;32(3):183–93.
10. Krakauer M, Botero JF, Lavalle-González FJ, et al. A review of flash glucose monitoring in type 2 diabetes. Diabetol Metab Syndr 2021;13:42.

11. Welsh JB, Gao P, Derdzinski M, et al. Accuracy, utilization, and effectiveness comparisons of different continuous glucose monitoring systems. Diabetes Technology Ther 2019;21(3):128–32.

12. Carlson A, Mullen D, Bergenstal RM, et al. Clinical use of continuous glucose monitoring in adults with type 2 diabetes. Diabetes Technology Ther 2017;19(2):S4–11.

13. Christiansen MP, Klaff LJ, Brazg R, et al. A prospective multicenter evaluation of the accuracy of a novel implanted continuous glucose sensor: PRECISE II. Diabetes Technology Ther 2018;20(3):197–206.

14. Dexcom. Welcome to Dexcom CLARITY, your diabetes management application. 2015-2021. Available at: https://clarity.dexcom.com/. June 28, 2021.

15. Abbott. Discover the mobile apps. 2021. Available at: https://www.freestyle. abbott/us-en/products/freestyle-libre-app.html?utm_source=Google&utm_ medium=SEM&utm_campaign=Brand&utm_content=App&gclid=Cj0KCQjw5u WGBhCTARIsAL70sLIe9qMi7eZ34HIVhR_JUf9B1biV68QtBgQT3UES1u2R7UJN AI0Ty7MaAjTLEALw_wcB&gclsrc=aw.ds. June 28, 2021.

16. Medtronic. About your diabetes with CareLink Reports. 2021. Available at: https:// www.medtronicdiabetes.com/products/carelink-personal-diabetes-software. June 28, 2021.

17. Senseonics, Inc. Eversense Health Care Provider User Guides. 2019. Available at: https://resources.eversensediabetes.com/resources/hcp. June 28, 2021.

18. Senseonics, Inc. Eversense Continuous Glucose Monitoring System Data Management System (DMS) Pro User Guide. 2019. Accessed June 28, 2021.

19. Radermecker RP, Scheen AJ. Continuous subcutaneous insulin infusion with short-acting insulin analogues or human regular insulin: efficacy, safety, quality of life, and cost-effectiveness. Diabetes Metab Res Rev 2004;20(3):178–88.

20. Paldus B, Lee MH, O'Neal DN. Insulin pumps in general practice. Aust Prescr 2018;41(6):186–90.

21. McAdams BH, Rizvi AA. An overview of insulin pumps and glucose sensors for the generalist. J Clin Med 2016;5(1):5.

22. Garg S, Moser E, Dain MP, et al. Clinical experience with insulin glargine in type 1 diabetes. Diabetes Technol Ther 2010;12(11):835–46.

23. American Diabetes Association. 7. Diabetes technology: standards of medical care in diabetes—2021. Am Diabetes Assoc Diabetes Care 2021;44(Supplement 1):S85–99.

24. Yeh HC, Brown TT, Maruthur N, et al. Comparative effectiveness and safety of methods of insulin delivery and glucose monitoring for diabetes mellitus: a systematic review and meta-analysis. Ann Intern Med 2012;157(5):336–47.

25. Gross TM, Kayne D, King A, et al. A bolus calculator is an effective means of controlling postprandial glycemia in patients on insulin pump therapy. Diabetes Technol Ther 2003;5(3):365–9.

26. Mehta SN, Quinn N, Volkening LK, et al. Impact of carbohydrate counting on glycemic control in children with type 1 diabetes. Diabetes Care 2009;32(6):1014–6.

27. Bell KJ, Smart CE, Steil GM, et al. Impact of fat, protein, and glycemic index on postprandial glucose control in type 1 diabetes: implications for intensive diabetes management in the continuous glucose monitoring era. Diabetes Care 2015;38(6):1008–15.

28. van der Hoogt M, van Dyk JC, Dolman RC, et al. Protein and fat meal content increase insulin requirement in children with type 1 diabetes: role of duration of diabetes. J Clin Transl Endocrinol 2017;10:15–21.

29. Lopez PE, Smart CE, McElduff P, et al. Optimizing the combination insulin bolus split for a high-fat, high-protein meal in children and adolescents using insulin pump therapy. Diabet Med 2017;34(10):1380–4.

30. O'Connell MA, Gilbertson HR, Donath SM, et al. Optimizing postprandial glyce-mia in pediatric patients with type 1 diabetes using insulin pump therapy: impact of glycemic index and prandial bolus type. Diabetes Care 2008;31(8):1491–5.

31. Steineck I, Ranjan A, Nørgaard K, et al. Sensor-augmented insulin pumps and hy-poglycemia prevention in type 1 diabetes. J Diabetes Sci Technol 2017;11(1):50–8.

32. Automated Insulin Delivery: Easy Enough to Use in Primary Care? Michael Heile, Betty Hollstegge, Laura Broxterman, Albert Cai. Kelly CloseClinical Diabetes Dec 2020;38(5):474–85.

33. Hermanides J, Nørgaard K, Bruttomesso D, et al. Sensor-augmented pump ther-apy lowers HbA(1c) in suboptimally controlled type 1 diabetes; a randomized controlled trial. Diabet Med 2011;28(10):1158–67.

34. User Guide Omnipod Dash Handbook. 2020. Available at: https://www.omnipod. com/sites/default/files/2021-04/Omnipod-DASH_User-Guide_English.pdf. June 29 2021.

35. Forlenza GP, Buckingham BA, Brown SA, et al. First outpatient evaluation of a tube-less automated insulin delivery system with customizable glucose targets in chil-dren and adults with type 1 diabetes. Diabetes Technol Ther 2021;23(6):410–24.

36. U. S Food and Drug Administration. The artificial pancreas device system. Avail-able at: https://www.Fda.gov/medical-devices/consumerproduct/artificial-pancrease-devicesystem Accessed June 17 2021.

37. MiniMed 770G System-P160017/S076. 2020. Available at: https://www.fda.gov/ medical-devices/recently-approved-devices/minimed-770g-system-p160017s076. June 21 2021.

38. Medtronic. MiniMed 770G System User Guide. 2020. Available at: https://www. medtronicdiabetes.com/sites/default/files/library/download-library/user-guides/ MiniMed_770G_System_User_Guide.pdf. June 21 2021.

39. Medtronic. MiniMed 670G System User Guide. 2017. Available at: https://www. medtronicdiabetes.com/sites/default/files/library/download-library/user-guides/ MiniMed-670G-System-User-Guide.pdf. July 3 2021.

40. Bergenstal RM, Garg S, Weinzimer SA, et al. Safety of a hybrid closed-loop insu-lin delivery system in patients with type 1 diabetes. JAMA 2016;316:1407–8.

41. Tandem. T:slim X2 Insulin Pump with Control – IQ Technology User Guide. Available at: https://www.tandemdiabetes.com/docs/default-source/product-documents/ t-slim-x2-insulin-pump/aw-1004379_d_user-guide-tslim-x2-control-iq-7-3-mgd-artwork-web.pdf?sfvrsn=18a507d7_60. June 29 2021.

42. Tandem. The t: connect Mobile App. 2021. Available at: https://www. tandemdiabetes.com/providers/products/tconnect-mobile-app. 29 June 29 2021.

43. Tandem. T:slim X2 Insulin Pump with Basal – IQ Technology User Guide. Available at: https://www.tandemdiabetes.com/docs/default-source/product-documents/t-slim-x2-insulin-pump/aw-1006684_c-user-guide-tslim-x2-basal-iq-6-4-mmoll-artwork-web.pdf?sfvrsn=eeb230d7_139. June 29 2021.

44. 120-LB: Early Real-World Hypoglycemia Outcomes with Use of the Tandem Basal-IQ Technology System, JORDAN E. PINSKER, KRISTIN N. CASTORINO, SCOTT A. LEAS, and STEPHANIE HABIF

45. Brown SA, Kovatchev BP, Raghinaru D, et al. iDCL Trial research Group. Six-month randomized, multicenter trial of close-loop control in type 1 diabetes. N Engl J Med 2019;381:1707–17.

46. Companion Medical. Inpen system instructions for use. Available at: https://www. companionmedical.com/guides/inpen-user-guide.pdf. June 28 2021.

47. Cui L, Schroeder PR, Sack PA. Inpatient and outpatient technologies to assist in the management of insulin dosing. Clin Diabetes 2020;38(5):462–73.

Inpatient Diabetes Management

Sumera Ahmed, MD, BC-ADM[a],*, Joseph Patrick Styers, PharmD, BCPS, BCCCP[b]

KEYWORDS

- Inpatient diabetes management • Inpatient treatment • Discharge planning
- Insulin in hospital

KEY POINTS

- Diabetes management in the inpatient setting is dynamic and requires coordinated care by a dedicated and specialized team.
- Basal-Bolus (Prandial)-correctional insulin regimen that is weight-eGFR (Estimated Glomerular Filtration Rate) based is preferred in the hospital setting.
- Hypoglycemia is the main adverse drug reaction and should be actively prevented, promptly treated, and tracked for systems improvements.
- Discharge planning should begin as soon as the patient stabilizes and a multidisciplinary team should be used to ensure continuity of care and address barriers to adherence.
- Advances in outpatient diabetes treatment technologies require special attention, training, and policies to support continued use in the hospital setting.

INTRODUCTION

Diabetes is a chronic disease affecting 34.2 million people in the United States as per the 2020 National Diabetes Statistics Report.[1] People with diabetes who require hospitalization are at higher risk for adverse outcomes due to hyperglycemia, hypoglycemia, and glycemic variability.[2] This article will review glycemic targets in the hospital, and insulin dosing, including special situations such as steroid-induced hyperglycemia, perioperative care, and parenteral and enteral nutrition (EN). This article will discuss glycemic adverse events, discharge planning and the role of technology in the inpatient setting.

DISCUSSION

The American Diabetes Association (ADA) defines hyperglycemia as blood glucose (BG) of more than 140 mg/dL (7.8 mmol/L).[2] There are 3 types of hyperglycemia seen during hospitalization as shown in **Box 1**.

---

[a] Primary Care Department, Diabetes Fellowship, Touro University College of Osteopathic Medicine, 1310 Club Drive, Vallejo, CA 94592, USA; [b] NorthBay Healthcare, 1200 B Gale Wilson Boulevard, Fairfield, CA 94533, USA
* Corresponding author.
E-mail address: Sahmed21@touro.edu

Prim Care Clin Office Pract 49 (2022) 339–349
https://doi.org/10.1016/j.pop.2021.11.006
0095-4543/22/© 2021 Elsevier Inc. All rights reserved.

Box 1
Types of hyperglycemia in hospitalized patients

Known history of diabetes

Existing, but unrecognized or undiagnosed diabetes

Stress hyperglycemia

The types of hyperglycemia can be differentiated by ordering an A1c on admission. A1c $\geq$ 6.5% indicates a prior history of diabetes (diagnosed or undiagnosed).[2] A1c $\leq$ 6.4% indicates stress hyperglycemia, although diabetes cannot be completely excluded, and an oral glucose tolerance test may be considered after discharge.[3] Hyperglycemia on admission and during hospitalization signifies poor clinical outcome, increased mortality, longer length of stay, and complications.[4,5] As such it is imperative that adequate BG control be an aim in the inpatient setting.

Glycemic Targets

The ADA recommends insulin therapy in treating persistent hyperglycemia when BG is more than 180 mg/dL. The ADA, American Association of Clinical Endocrinology (AACE) and Endocrine Society recommend target BG of 140 to 180 mg/dL for most of the critically ill and noncritically ill, nonpregnant adult patients.[2,6,7] Lower targets of 110 to 140 mg/dL can be considered in certain patients who are postcardiac surgery provided hypoglycemia is avoided.[2,7] Higher targets may be acceptable in patients with severe comorbidities and in terminally ill patients.[2,7]

Admission Checklists for Noncritically Ill Patients

When providers admit patients to the hospital, consider a checklist when placing admitting orders for patients with diabetes. See **Box 2**.

Box 2
Checklist for admitting orders

- Measure BG on admission
- Obtain A1c if BG greater than 140 mg/dL or if patient has a known history of diabetes and A1c result within last 90 days is not available[2]
- Identify and document type of diabetes
- Review home medications and level of glucose control if preexisting diabetes
- If BG greater than 140 mg/dL or h/o diabetes, order finger stick BG monitoring based on nutritional pattern[2]
  - If on diet – q ACHS (before meals and at bedtime)
  - If NPO (nothing by mouth) or on tube feeding or total parenteral nutrition – every 4 to 6 hours
  - 3 AM check (at the first initiation of insulin, patients at risk for hypoglycemia, or glycemic variability)[3]
- Diet – Carbohydrate-consistent and calorie-restricted diet[3]
- Discharge planning to be initiated early in hospitalization to ensure adequate time in learning skills in the home management of diabetes

---

Management

ADA, AACE, and Endocrine Society guidelines recommend insulin in the management of hyperglycemia in the hospital setting and the sole use of sliding-scale insulin is strongly discouraged.[2,6–8] Insulin can be administered by intravenous (IV) and subcutaneous (SC) route in the hospital. Regular insulin is given as a continuous infusion or "IV drip" peaks immediately in 2 minutes and has a half-life of 5 minutes.[9] Thus, when IV infusion is discontinued, plasma insulin levels drop rapidly within about 20 minutes.[10] IV insulin is used in the critical care settings in the treatment of diabetic emergencies—diabetic ketoacidosis (DKA) and hyperglycemic hyperosmolar state. Other indications whereby IV insulin is preferred in the hospital setting are surgical and postoperative care, prolonged NPO, labor and delivery, and glucose toxicity with persistent hyperglycemia despite adequate basal-bolus regimen as seen with steroid use. Insulin given via the SC route exists as hexamers, 6 molecules of insulin around a zinc molecule, and hexamer molecules cannot cross the capillary membrane.[3,10] This forms the depot after an SC injection. The hexamers are broken down into dimers and monomers which then cross the capillary membrane into the bloodstream.

Components of Subcutaneous Insulin Regimen

The components of an effective SC insulin regimen in the inpatient setting consist of basal insulin, prandial or nutritional insulin, and correctional insulin. Basal insulin is to meet the heightened metabolic requirements that are seen during hospitalizations. This is usually 50% of the total daily dose (TDD). Glargine insulin once daily at bedtime is preferred.[10] Detemir insulin can be used once or twice daily and NPH insulin can be used twice daily (2/3 in AM and 1/3 in PM). NPH increases the risk of hypoglycemia due to its peak effect at 4 to 6 hours, especially in patients who may be required to be kept NPO for procedures and other indications.[3] Premixed insulins (70/30, 75/25, 50/50) are not recommended in the inpatient setting due to higher rates of hypoglycemia.[3] Prandial insulin, also known as nutritional or bolus insulin, is used for the expected hyperglycemia with the intake of carbohydrates with meals or with enteral or parenteral nutrition. This is usually the remaining 50% of the TDD (split between 3 meals) but may be less in hospitalized patients due to reduced oral intake. Analog insulins (Lispro, Aspart, or Glulisine) are preferred over Regular insulin as they have less risk of hypoglycemia.[3] Prandial insulin should be given before each meal. Specific instructions to hold the dose if the patient is not eating and reduce the dose by 50% if oral intake is 50% or less should be written in the orders. If the patient's anticipated meal consumption is unknown, the dose may be given directly following a meal. It is critical to coordinate the nutritional dose of insulin close to meal intake to avoid hyperglycemia with delayed dose, and hypoglycemia due to insulin-food mismatch. Correctional doses are given to correct for unexpected hyperglycemia, and the type of insulin should match the insulin type used for prandial dosing. This correction dose is added to prandial dose insulin and is given as one injection.

Calculation of insulin doses – When starting insulin, the patients' renal function (GFR), age and comorbidities, BMI, type of diabetes, and control before hospitalization (A1c) should be taken into consideration.[3,10] There are 3 suggested methods to calculate TDD insulin:

a. Weight-GFR based (preferred in most cases)
b. Patient's home dose (which can often be unreliable)
c. Based on IV insulin infusion during transition from IV to SC insulin

Weight-GFR based insulin regimen is the preferred method of calculation. See **Table 1**. Patients who have only been on oral agents and have an A1c <7%, or patients

Table 1
Weight-GFR based total daily dose insulin calculation

	Type 1 Diabetes	Type 2 Diabetes
Normal renal function[10]	0.4 U/kg/d	0.5 U/kg/d
Impaired renal function[10]	GFR 10–50 mL/min - 0.3 U/kg/d	GFR 10–50 mL/min - 0.3 U/kg/d
	GFR<10 mL/min - 0.2 U/kg/d	GFR<10 mL/min - 0.2 U/kg/d
Age>70 and comorbidities[10]	0.3 U/kg/d	0.3 U/kg/d
BMI<19[10]	0.3 U/kg/d	0.3 U/kg/d
A1c - 7%–7.9%[3]	0.2–0.3 U/kg/d	0.2–0.3 U/kg/d
A1c - 8%–9.9% or BG 140–200[3]	0.4 U/kg/d	0.4 U/kg/d
A1c ≥ 10% or BG 200–400[3]	0.5 unit/kg/d	0.5 unit/kg/d

Data from Refs [3,10]

with newly diagnosed diabetes who are insulin-naïve can be started on correctional insulin doses alone. If BG is consistently over 140 mg/dL, basal insulin should be initiated at 0.1 U/kg/d[3,10].

Most providers tend to continue home doses of insulin on admission. This can be considered if patients' diabetes is well controlled with no hypoglycemia at home on their regimen. As oral intake may be reduced during hospitalization due to general dislike of "hospital food" it is recommended to decrease prandial insulin initially by 25% to 50% to prevent hypoglycemia.[3] It is important to assess and modify insulin doses on a daily or more frequent basis as insulin requirements can change due to change in a patient's clinical condition, severity of illness, glucose trajectory, oral intake, and dynamic nature of hospital care.[11] A coordinated diabetes management team consisting of physicians, pharmacists, nurses, certified diabetes educators, and dieticians is essential for providing high-quality care to patients with diabetes.

Oral Agents and Noninsulin Injectables

The AACE and Endocrine Society do not recommend the use of oral antihyperglycemic agents (OADs) in the hospital.[7,11] Although ADA recommended against the use of OADs in earlier guidelines, the recent 2021 ADA guidelines state that, in certain circumstances, oral agents may be continued in hospitalized patients.[2,12] DPP4-inhibitors, Linagliptin and GLP-1 RA, Dulaglutide have shown potential effectiveness in selected groups of hospitalized patients in Randomized Controlled Trials.[2] Saxagliptin and Alogliptin should be avoided in patients with heart failure based on FDA bulletin.[2] Metformin is generally held for 48 hours after IV contrast injection and discontinued for GFR less than 60 mL/min/1.73m2, hypoxic states, and patients with liver disease.[3] Evidence supports continuing metformin therapy in patients with appropriate kidney function who have received one dose of iodinated contrast.[13] A paradigm shift has occurred about the risk of MALA (metformin-associated lactic acidosis) versus the benefit of metformin, and many experts are weighing in to push the scales toward encouraging metformin therapy and acknowledging that the risk of MALA is very low.[14] Sulfonylureas should be discontinued in patients with acute kidney injury and chronic kidney disease and patients who are NPO.[3] Pioglitazone should be avoided in patients with a history of heart failure and edema.[3]

Adverse Inpatient Events

Improper diabetes management may cause hypoglycemia, an adverse drug reaction that may lead to fatal outcomes. Inpatient mortality and length of stay are both increased for patients who experience hypoglycemia during admission.[15] Level 1 hypoglycemia is defined as a BG concentration 54 to 70 mg/dL, level 2 as less than 54 mg/dL, and level 3 as a hypoglycemia event that caused significantly reduced functioning and required intervention from another person.[16] Patients experiencing level 2 or level 3 hypoglycemia may experience neurologic symptoms, and prolonged time at these blood sugar levels may cause seizures, coma, or death.

Inpatient providers can leverage the strengths of the electronic health record to streamline hypoglycemia treatment in the hospital. Predetermined order sets for insulin can be designed to include oral glucose, IV dextrose, and glucagon (with parameters) for administration to treat acute hyperglycemia. Computerized physician order entry (CPOE) can provide standardized sliding scale insulin orders that are agreed on within the institution. CPOE-provided regimens for hyperglycemia have been demonstrated to increase time at target BG while not increasing the risk of hypoglycemia.[2] Similar results are seen in critically ill patients with a computerized insulin infusion protocol integrated into patient care using CPOE.[17] An institution could also adopt an electronic glucose management system, a software system designed to aid providers in decision-making which has shown to decrease time in hypoglycemia.[18]

Monitoring adverse drug events and reactions is a top patient safety priority for hospitals. The electronic medical record should be used to gather data on adverse drug events in patients with diabetes, particularly those involving hypoglycemia. Nurses, physicians, and patients may underreport adverse reactions such as hypoglycemia, but the events can be elucidated from a patient's chart using techniques such as the Institute for Healthcare Improvement's Global Trigger Tool.[19,20] This tool suggests setting up "triggers" to alert for a possible adverse drug event. Examples of triggers include any glucose level less than 50 mg/dL or an IV push of dextrose 50%. A medication safety officer can then review for the administration of antihyperglycemics. Trends can be analyzed for improvements on a systems level.

SPECIAL SITUATIONS
Steroid-Induced Hyperglycemia

Steroid-induced hyperglycemia refers to hyperglycemia (BG > 180 mg/dL) in the setting of steroid use and can occur in patients with and without preexisting diabetes.[3,21] Steroids cause primarily postprandial hyperglycemia due to the suppression of insulin secretion, increased gluconeogenesis, and insulin resistance.[21] Recommendations for the management of steroid-induced hyperglycemia are based on expert opinion and observational studies. NPH insulin or a modified Basal Bolus regimen can be considered. NPH insulin can be added once a day in the morning for patients on oral prednisone once daily in the morning.[21] A suggested the method of calculating starting NPH insulin dose is basing it on the dose of prednisone. For patients on prednisone 10 mg/d, start at 0.1 units/kg/d with dose increased by 0.1 units/kg/d for every 10 mg increase in prednisone dose up to 0.4 units/kg/d for prednisone 40 mg or more per day.[22] Modified basal-bolus regimen at 30% basal and 70% bolus or prandial insulin (instead of 50/50 regimen) can be considered especially for patients on long-acting(dexamethasone) or multiple daily doses of steroids (IV hydrocortisone or methylprednisolone). Basal insulin can include insulin glargine or detemir insulin.[21] A randomized controlled trial that compared efficacy and safety of insulin glargine versus NPH insulin as basal insulin for the treatment of steroid-induced hyperglycemia showed that both were equally effective.[23]

Perioperative Care

The ADA recommends target BG 80 to 180 mg/dL during the perioperative period as tighter control does not improve outcomes and is associated with more hypoglycemia.[2] BG should be monitored every 2 to 4 hours when the patient is NPO, and correctional rapid or short-acting insulin be given every 4 to 6 hours as needed.[2] Long-acting insulin should be reduced to 75% to 80% of the dose on the morning of or night before surgery.[2] Reduce NPH insulin to 50% of dose on the morning of surgery.[2] It is critical that long-acting insulin not be held for patients with type 1 diabetes to avoid the precipitation of DKA. OADs are to be held on the morning of surgery and until oral intake is resumed.[2] IV insulin is preferred for patients undergoing major surgeries or surgeries lasting over 3 to 4 hours.[3,10] Although the GLOLIA study showed that the addition of low-dose liraglutide to insulin achieved better glycemic control during the perioperative period, further RCT studies are needed, and current ADA guidelines do not recommend the continuation of GLP-1 RA at this time in the hospital setting.[24]

Transition from Intravenous to Subcutaneous Insulin

Transitioning from IV to SC insulin must be conducted when patients are hemodynamically stable and tolerating at least 50% of their diet.[3] As it takes 2 hours to build an adequate depot of any SC, long-acting insulin must be injected at least 2 to 4 hours before stopping the insulin infusion.[10] Determine total infusion amount for the last 6 hours, preferably overnight when the patient is not eating. Multiply the 6-hour infusion amount by 4 to determine the projected 24-hour insulin requirement. Use 60%–80% of this amount for the long-acting basal insulin dose. Add 20%–40% of the calculated 24-hours dose as prandial (bolus insulin) with each meal.[3,10]

Total Parenteral Nutrition and Enteral Feeding

Continuous EN places patients at risk for hyperglycemia due to the stress reaction of an acute illness along with the theoretic inhibition of incretin hormones as a result of continuous feeding.[25] For these patients, continue the basal dose and add nutritional coverage as rapid-acting insulin every 4 hours or regular insulin every 6 hours, calculating the dose as 1 unit of insulin for every 10 to 15 g of carbohydrates in the formulation.[2] For patients on bolus or cyclic feeding, timing and formulation of nutritional insulin will need to be adjusted appropriately. Correctional insulin should also be provided as needed. Diabetes-specific formulations to prevent hyperglycemia (eg, Glucerna) are controversial, and current ASPEN guidelines do not recommend using them.[26]

Parenteral nutrition (PN) also requires interventions to avoid hyperglycemia in patients with diabetic. More than 50% of patients on parenteral nutrition in the hospital experience hyperglycemia, which is associated with increased mortality.[25] Hyperglycemia can be prevented by lowering the dextrose content and calories in the PN. Adding EN to PN if tolerated is also shown to lower glucose concentrations and reduce insulin resistance.[25] For the treatment of hyperglycemia requiring significant SC correctional insulin, 1 unit of insulin per 10 g of dextrose should be added to the bag and correctional insulin continued.[26] This strategy theoretically lowers the risk of hypoglycemia when the PN is paused or discontinued, avoids injections, and requires less nursing input but supporting evidence is weak and there is concern about insulin stability and adsorption to the bag.[25,27] Close monitoring and frequent treatment adjustments are needed for acutely ill patients receiving PN.

Technology

Technologies used to improve outpatient diabetes management continue to advance but there can be confusion about who should manage the devices when a patient is admitted to the hospital. Insulin pumps, continuous glucose monitors, and related devices are often managed at home by the patient. Hospital staff unfamiliar with these devices may be uncomfortable, posing a medication safety risk.

Patients admitted with a continuous SC insulin infusion (CSII or insulin pump) raise the question of whether or not to continue the CSII while receiving inpatient care. The 2021 ADA Standards of Medical Care in Diabetes offer an expert consensus stating patients may continue to use their pumps if physically and cognitively able.[2] A large cohort study in Arizona showed improved safety outcomes in patients using their own CSII during inpatient stay.[28] Cases of hyperglycemia and hypoglycemia were significantly lower in the "pump on" group. Patients who manage their insulin pump at home tend to be more familiar with its workings than the inpatient physicians and nurses. A collaboration between the patient and staff may be beneficial when developing a care plan. Consider implementing a signed agreement detailing the responsibilities of both the patient and staff to ensure clarity. A thorough record of insulin type, pump model, and settings should be obtained and made easily accessible in the electronic health record.[29] Hospital policies and protocols should be developed, and staff trained accordingly.

Inpatient use of an insulin pump is not always appropriate, such as in cases of critical illness, prolonged surgery, diabetic emergency, device malfunction, or in patients with cognitive or physical impairment.[29] In such a case, the pump should be disabled, and an appropriate IV insulin therapy or basal-bolus regimen should be started. When transitioning back to the pump, the IV infusion should overlap by approximately 2 hours to allow sufficient maturation of a SC depot of insulin.[29]

Real-time continuous glucose monitoring (CGM) devices sample interstitial BG as a surrogate for plasma glucose. These devices have been poorly studied in the inpatient setting, although data show an improvement in A1c and a decrease in hypoglycemia in the outpatient setting. Some small studies demonstrate improved detection of hypoglycemic events with inpatient CGM over fingerstick glucose testing, but this did not translate to improved time in target glucose.[30,31] The COVID-19 pandemic spurred interest in noninvasive remote monitoring systems including CGM utilization. CGM is not currently FDA approved for inpatient monitoring, but it was allowed temporarily during the emergency to conserve personal protective equipment and better monitor patients.[32]

Discharge Planning/Care Transitions

Inpatient diabetes education requires a multidisciplinary effort beginning as early as possible following patient stabilization.[2] Initial evaluation of the patient's ability to self-manage is essential to identify patient-specific barriers to self-care. A patient's insurance status, financial ability, family support, personal motivation, and health literacy are all essential components to a successful education program. Diabetes education must reinforce the importance of self-management and highlight personal nutrition, glucometer use, hypoglycemia identification and management, insulin or other pharmaceutical administration, and medical waste disposal.[33,34] Patients who are preoccupied with their acute illness and with the stress of the inpatient setting are particularly likely to be unable to retain teaching,[33] requiring consistent and repeated reinforcement of management goals.

Importance must be placed on gathering an accurate and complete medication history. The Joint Commission has named medication reconciliation as one of its 2021 National Patient Safety Goals.[35] Confirming dose, compliance, and most recent administration is important for all medications but especially so for high-risk medications such as insulin. A medication list of outpatient medications should be gathered and reconciled with inpatient orders to reduce the frequency of medication errors.[36] On discharge, the patient should be provided with an updated list of current medications in their discharge paperwork. A clinical staff member should review the medication list with the patient at the time of discharge.[36]

Choice of discharge treatment must be tailored to the patient. The decision to initiate an outpatient insulin regimen should take into account the patient's cognitive abilities, dexterity, and willingness to perform injections and fingersticks.[33] For visually impaired patients, insulin pens may be preferred over vials as it is easier to read the dose than on a syringe.[33] Patients without stable housing may not be able to store medications that require refrigeration.

Due to the high cost of diabetes medications and supplies, insurance issues should be identified early in the admission. Inpatient formularies may not align with insurance formularies so medication changes may be required. Case managers, social workers, nurses, and pharmacists can assist in determining coverage and confirming availability and copays at the outpatient pharmacy before discharge. Supplies such as testing strips and glucose monitors should also be prescribed to a pharmacy and checked to ensure the correct brand and to allow for insurance coverage.

Follow-up appointments and transportation also need to be arranged to ensure the continuum of care. ADA guidelines recommend every patient with hyperglycemia have a follow-up appointment within 1 month of discharge or within 1 to 2 weeks if medications have changed or glucose levels are uncontrolled.[2]

SUMMARY

Diabetes management in the inpatient setting is dynamic and requires coordinated care by a dedicated and specialized team. Care should be individualized and patient-centric. National guidelines recommend a glycemic target of 140 to 180 for most hospitalized patients with some exceptions. Insulin is preferred in the treatment of diabetes with avoidance of hypoglycemia and hyperglycemia. Discharge planning should begin as soon as the patient stabilizes and use a multidisciplinary team to ensure the continuum of care and address barriers to adherence. Advances in outpatient diabetes treatment technologies require special attention, training, and policies to support continued use in the hospital setting.

CLINICS CARE POINTS

- Documenting the type of diabetes in patients' charts is important to ensure basal or long-acting insulin is not discontinued in patients with Type 1 diabetes.

- The ADA, AACE, and Endocrine Society recommend a target BG of 140 to 180 mg/dL for most of the critically ill and noncritically ill, nonpregnant adult patients in the hospital.

- Calculate the total daily insulin dose based on the type of diabetes, eGFR, age, A1c on admission, BMI, and starting doses can range from 0.2 to 0.5 units/kg/d.

- The IHI's Global Trigger Tool can retrospectively identify hypoglycemic events to allow for systematic review.

- Outpatient diabetes medications and supplies can be prohibitively expensive. Copays should be confirmed with the outpatient pharmacy before discharge if there is a question of coverage.

- Allow patients to continue to use their insulin pump while inpatient if they are cognitively and physically able and the hospital has clear policies and procedures around the matter.

DISCLOSURE

S. Ahmed is on the advisory committee for DiabetesWise Pro. J.P. Styers has nothing to disclose.

REFERENCES

1. Centers for Disease Control and Prevention. National diabetes Statistics Report, 2020. Atlanta (GA): Centers for Disease Control and Prevention, U.S. Dept of Health and Human Services; 2020.
2. American Diabetes Association. 15. Diabetes Care in the Hospital: Standards of Medical Care in Diabetes-2021. Diabetes Care 2021;44(Suppl 1):S211–20.
3. Khazai NB, Hamdy O. Inpatient Diabetes Management in the Twenty-First Century. Endocrinol Metab Clin North Am 2016;45(4):875–94.
4. Umpierrez GE, Isaacs SD, Bazargan N, et al. Hyperglycemia: an independent marker of in-hospital mortality in patients with undiagnosed diabetes. J Clin Endocrinol Metab 2002;87(3):978–82.
5. Furnary AP, Wu Y. Clinical effects of hyperglycemia in the cardiac surgery population: the Portland Diabetic Project. Endocr Pract 2006;12(Suppl 3):22–6.
6. Available at: https://pro.aace.com/disease-state-resources/diabetes/guidelines. Accessed on July 18, 2021.
7. Umpierrez GE, Hellman R, Korytkowski MT, et al. Management of hyperglycemia in hospitalized patients in non-critical care setting: an endocrine society clinical practice guideline. J Clin Endocrinol Metab 2012;97(1):16–38.
8. Available at: https://www.endocrinepractice.org/article/S1530-891X(20)43462-7/fulltext. Accessed on July 18, 2021.
9. Guerra SM, Kitabchi AE. Comparison of the effectiveness of various routes of insulin injection: insulin levels and glucose response in normal subjects. J Clin Endocrinol Metab 1976;42(5):869–74.
10. Hardee S, Tanenberg RJ, The Diabetes Blue Book-Practical Inpatient Management of Adults with Diabetes and Hyperglycemia, 7th edition, Aug 2016.
11. Moghissi ES, Korytkowski MT, DiNardo M, et al. American Association of Clinical Endocrinologists and American Diabetes Association consensus statement on inpatient glycemic control. Diabetes Care 2009;32(6):1119–31.
12. American Diabetes Association. 15. Diabetes Care in the Hospital: Standards of Medical Care in Diabetes-2020. Diabetes Care 2020;43(Suppl 1):S193–202.
13. Goergen SK, Rumbold G, Compton G, et al. Systematic review of current guidelines, and their evidence base, on risk of lactic acidosis after administration of contrast medium for patients receiving metformin. Radiology 2010;254(1):261–9.
14. Salvatore T, Pafundi PC, Marfella R, et al. Metformin lactic acidosis: Should we still be afraid? Diabetes Res Clin Pract 2019;157:107879.
15. Borzì V, Frasson S, Gussoni G, et al. Risk factors for hypoglycemia in patients with type 2 diabetes, hospitalized in internal medicine wards: Findings from the FADOI-DIAMOND study. Diabetes Res Clin Pract 2016;115:24–30.
16. Agiostratidou G, Anhalt H, Ball D, et al. Standardizing clinically meaningful outcome measures beyond HbA1c for Type 1 diabetes: a consensus report of the american association of clinical endocrinologists, the American Association of Diabetes Educators, the American Diabetes Association, the Endocrine Society, JDRF International, The Leona M. and Harry B. Helmsley Charitable Trust, the Pediatric Endocrine Society, and the T1D Exchange. Diabetes Care 2017;40(12):1622–30.

17. Boord JB, Sharifi M, Greevy RA, et al. Computer-based insulin infusion protocol improves glycemia control over manual protocol. J Am Med Inform Assoc 2007;14(3):278–87.
18. Cruz P. Inpatient hypoglycemia: the challenge remains. J Diabetes Sci Technol 2020;14(3):560–6.
19. Adler L, Denham CR, McKeever M, et al. Global trigger tool: implementation basics. J Patient Saf 2008;4(4):245–9.
20. Classen DC, Lloyd RC, Provost L, et al. Development and Evaluation of the Institute for Healthcare Improvement Global Trigger Tool. J Patient Saf 2008;4(3): 169–77.
21. Mathioudakis N; Dungan K; Baldwin D; Korytkowski M; Reider J - Managing Diabetes and Hyperglycemia in the hospital setting-Clinician's Guide –Boris Draznin.
22. Clore JN, Thurby-Hay L. Glucocorticoid-induced hyperglycemia. Endocr Pract 2009;15(5):469–74.
23. Ruiz de Adana MS, Colomo N, Maldonado-Araque C, et al. Randomized clinical trial of the efficacy and safety of insulin glargine vs. NPH insulin as basal insulin for the treatment of glucocorticoid induced hyperglycemia using continuous glucose monitoring in hospitalized patients with type 2 diabetes and respiratory disease. Diabetes Res Clin Pract 2015;110(2):158–65.
24. Makino H, Tanaka A, Asakura K, et al. Addition of low-dose liraglutide to insulin therapy is useful for glycaemic control during the peri-operative period: effect of glucagon-like peptide-1 receptor agonist therapy on glycaemic control in patients undergoing cardiac surgery (GLOLIA study). Diabet Med 2019;36(12): 1621–8.
25. Drincic AT, Knezevich JT, Akkireddy P. Nutrition and HYPERGLYCEMIA management in the inpatient Setting (Meals on Demand, Parenteral, or Enteral Nutrition). Curr Diab Rep 2017;17(8). https://doi.org/10.1007/s11892-017-0882-3.
26. McMahon MM, Nystrom E, Braunschweig C, et al. N. clinical guidelines. J Parenter Enteral Nutr 2012;37(1):23–36.
27. McCulloch A, Bansiya V, Woodward JM. Addition of insulin to parenteral nutrition for control of hyperglycemia. J Parenter Enteral Nutr 2017. https://doi.org/10. 1177/0148607117722750. 014860711772275.
28. Cook CB, Beer KA, Seifert KM, et al. Transitioning insulin pump therapy from the outpatient to the inpatient setting: a review of 6 years' experience with 253 cases. J Diabetes Sci Technol 2012;6(5):995–1002.
29. Umpierrez GE, Klonoff DC. Diabetes technology update: use of insulin pumps and continuous glucose monitoring in the hospital. Diabetes Care 2018;41(8): 1579–89.
30. Levitt DL, Spanakis EK, Ryan KA, et al. Insulin pump and continuous glucose monitor initiation in hospitalized patients with Type 2 diabetes mellitus. Diabetes Technol Ther 2018;20(1):32–8.
31. Schaupp L, Donsa K, Neubauer KM, et al. Taking a closer look–continuous glucose monitoring in non-critically Ill hospitalized patients with type 2 diabetes mellitus under basal-bolus insulin therapy. Diabetes Technol Ther 2015;17(9):611–8.
32. U.S. Food and Drug Administration. Enforcement Policy for Non-Invasive Remote Monitoring Devices Used to Support Patient Monitoring During the Coronavirus Disease 2019 (COVID-19) Public Health Emergency (Revised). U.S. Food and Drug Administration. 2020. Available at: https://www.fda.gov/regulatory-information/search-fda-guidance-documents/enforcement-policy-non-invasive-remote-monitoring-devices-used-support-patient-monitoring-during. Accessed July 14, 2021.

33. Donihi AC. Practical Recommendations for Transitioning Patients with Type 2 Diabetes from Hospital to Home. Curr Diab Rep 2017;17(7):52.
34. Arnold P, Scheurer D, Dake AW, et al. Hospital Guidelines for Diabetes Management and the Joint Commission-American Diabetes Association Inpatient Diabetes Certification. Am J Med Sci 2016;351(4):333–41.
35. The Joint Commission. National patient safety Goals® effective January 2021 for the hospital program. 2021. Available at: https://www.jointcommission.org/standards/national-patient-safety-goals/hospital-national-patient-safety-goals/. Accessed July 16, 2021.
36. Kripalani S, Jackson AT, Schnipper JL, et al. Promoting effective transitions of care at hospital discharge: a review of key issues for hospitalists. J Hosp Med 2007;2(5):314–23.

Resources for Patients with Diabetes Mellitus

Beatriz Francesca Ramirez, MD

KEYWORDS

- Resources for patients with diabetes • Assistance • Insulin help
- Diabetes education • Tools for diabetes • Diabetes management
- Benefits for patients with diabetes

KEY POINTS

- Diabetes is a costly disease, and patients are often overwhelmed by both financial and quality-of-life demands, which renders them powerless to care for the disease.
- There are barriers inherent to patients that contribute to poor metabolic control, including adherence, beliefs, attitudes, knowledge, ethnicity/culture, language ability, financial resources, comorbidities, and social support. In addition, adherence to self-management is influenced by an individual's financial resources, beliefs and attitudes about the disease, and effectiveness of the treatment regimen.
- There are multiple resources available in the United States to help patients with these barriers. The clinician is responsible to seek the necessary knowledge regarding help available for the patients that they care for.
- A multidisciplinary team needs to be accessible to the provider so they can connect patients to the necessary services.

INTRODUCTION

Diabetes has reached epidemic proportions, and in United States, 34.2 million people have diabetes (10.5% of the US population), with 88 million people already in the prediabetic state (34.8% of the adult US population). The total direct and indirect estimated cost of diagnosed diabetes in the United States in 2017 was $327 billion.[1] Diabetes is a very expensive disease, and many patients do not have the necessary means to care for this condition.

Thanks to medical research we are undergoing an unprecedented explosion in the development of new treatments for patients with diabetes. There are multiple new drugs on the market as well as technology available to help them manage the disease. However, despite all these important advances, inadequate metabolic control continues.

Brody School of Medicine, East Carolina University, 600 Moye Boulevard, Greenville, NC 27834, USA
E-mail address: ramirezb@ecu.edu

Prim Care Clin Office Pract 49 (2022) 351–362
https://doi.org/10.1016/j.pop.2021.12.001
0095-4543/22/© 2021 Elsevier Inc. All rights reserved.
primarycare.theclinics.com

Multiple barriers interfere with the management of diabetes and prevent patients from achieving adequate glycemic control. Some obstacles intrinsic to patients include adherence, attitude, beliefs, and health literacy, which have a direct impact on how they care for themselves. Other influential factors include the patient's financial resources, comorbidities, and social support, among others.[2] Knowing what difficulties affect our patients will help us connect them to the appropriate resources.

It is the clinician's responsibility not only to be knowledgeable in the management of diabetes but also to help patients navigate this complex health care system. This responsibility involves learning about the different sources of assistance for their patients. The purpose of this article is to provide information on the different types of support offered at a national level. Help for patients with diabetes will depend on location; providers need to acquire knowledge about their local programs and reach out within their own communities to learn about different institutions and federally funded government programs that may be available to patients.

HISTORICAL BACKGROUND

In 1974, as diabetes became the fifth leading cause of death in the United States, Congress passed the National Diabetes Mellitus Research and Education Act.[3]

Funding increased immediately for basic research to determine the causes, cures, and means of preventing diabetes to encourage the translation of new knowledge into clinical practice and to promote the dissemination of information to diabetics and health care professionals.[3]

As the government's interest in diabetes grew, so too did the interests of the pharmaceutical and medical technology industries. They developed oral diabetic medicines, first marketed in the 1950s, as well as new insulins, lancets, syringes, glucose monitors, test strips, and insulin pumps, enabling diabetics to better and more effectively manage their blood glucose levels.[3]

Over the last century, insulin has evolved from poorly defined extracts of animal pancreata to pure and precisely controlled formulations that can be prescribed and administered with high accuracy and predictability of action.[4] Likewise, new oral and injectable antidiabetic agents have come to prominence, as data from clinical trials have shown that many of these drugs (sodium glucose co-transporter-2 inhibitors, glucagon-like peptide-1 receptor agonists) protect the heart and kidneys remarkably well.[5] In addition, continuous glucose monitoring devices and insulin pumps as well as a series of smart meters and insulin pens have revolutionized the way some patients are able to manage diabetes.

The reality is that not all patients have access to these resources. In 2019, as many as 14.5% of adults aged 18 to 64 years were uninsured in the United States. The percentage of uninsured adults who were uninsured because coverage was not affordable increased with age, from 66.8% among those aged 18 to 29 years to 80.9% among those aged 50 to 64 years.[6] In addition, it is well known that many of these uninsured patients will use the emergency departments for their primary care needs, creating an unnecessary burden to these services.

The field of diabetes has become increasingly complex at a time when there is a huge shortage of endocrinologists in the United States. Primary care providers are left to manage about 90% of patients with diabetes, and many of them lack the resources and time to devote to helping these very difficult patients.

Besides intensive training in diabetes management, the provider needs to be educated on the use of a team approach that includes certified diabetes educators, that is, nurses, dieticians, and pharmacists, plus supporting ophthalmologists, nephrologists, podiatrists, social workers, and psychologists. With these services in place, it will be much easier to overcome the barriers that prevent patients from achieving good diabetes control.

OVERCOMING OBSTACLES IN DIABETES SELF-MANAGEMENT

The obstacles that are inherent to patients include adherence, beliefs, attitudes, knowledge, ethnicity/culture, language ability, financial resources, comorbidities, and social support. Seven studies found that adherence to self-management is influenced by an individual's financial resources, beliefs and attitudes about the disease, and effectiveness of the treatment regimen.[7–12]

When patients look for information about diabetes, they can be easily overwhelmed by the number of documents available. They get information from social media (Twitter, Instagram, Tik Tok) newspapers, online, different organizations such as those found on Facebook, books, and different apps on their smartphones. However, as a clinician, it is important to direct our patients to good-quality and truthful information that can provide necessary education.

As George Bernard Shaw said, "Beware of false knowledge, it is more dangerous than ignorance."

DIABETES EDUCATION

Diabetes education can help to address issues with adherence, beliefs, and attitude toward the disease. Education cannot fall solely on the primary provider's shoulders. It is necessary to convince the patient to have a diabetes educator in their team of providers.

Diabetes Self-Management Education and Support

DSME or "Diabetes Self-Management Education" is an evidence-based service to help people with diabetes live longer and healthier lives. It is eligible for reimbursement by Medicare, many private health plans, and some state Medicaid agencies.[13]

DSME is supported by numerous studies that report associations between DSME and support and improved health. Diabetes Self-Management Education and Support (DSMES) services have been shown to have a positive impact on lifestyle changes, such as eating patterns and activity levels, ultimately leading to decreases in hemoglobin A1c levels, prevention or delay of diabetes complications, and improved quality of life.[14]

DSME is "the active, ongoing process of facilitating the knowledge, skill, and ability necessary for diabetes self-care." By combining DSME and DSMS (Diabetes Self-Management Support), services can "address the patient's health beliefs, cultural needs, current knowledge, physical limitations, emotional concerns, family support, financial status, medical history, health literacy, numeracy, and other factors that influence each person's ability to meet the challenges of self-management".[15]

To qualify for this program patients must have a diagnosis of type 1, type 2, or gestational diabetes and a referral from a qualified practitioner: physician (MD or DO), nurse practitioner, physician assistant, or advanced practice nurse.

Online Resources for Education

American Diabetes Association

American Diabetes Association (ADA) provides information on different diabetes programs based on patient's location. Some of these include the following:

- Diabetes risk test: a 60-second test to determine diabetes risk.
- Diabetes and COVID 19 education program.
- Diabetes food hub: diabetes-friendly recipes approved by ADA nutrition experts, daily meal planning.
- Living with type 2 diabetes program: a 12-month free program that provides information and support for patients who are newly diagnosed with type 2 diabetes.
- Insulin help: health education, medication management, and help with prescriptions.
- Diabetes education program locator: provides directory of ADA-approved Diabetes Education Programs across the nation.
- "Ask the Experts": a series designed to help people with diabetes confront commonly faced issues by providing a community where individuals can ask questions about diabetes and hear from others who may share similar experiences. The series includes information on diabetes management, health insurance information, meal preparation tips, physical activity advice, and interaction with experts knowledgeable about diabetes.
- Camp Sweeney: a 3-week summer program designed for children with diabetes. Patients must be 5 to 18 years old, and the cost is based on a sliding-scale fee.

All of these are available at www.diabetes.org/resources.[16]

American Heart Association

The American Heart Association and ADA have joined to provide "Know Diabetes by Heart" for type 2 diabetes and "Answers from the Experts" sessions on interesting diabetes topics. These educational resources are available to patients and providers for free. These can be found at https://www.heart.org/en/health-topics/diabetes/diabetes-tools–resources.[17]

Juvenile Diabetes Research Foundation

Online Diabetes Support Team by Juvenile Diabetes Research Foundation: specific for patients with type 1 diabetes, it provides health education, disease management, and virtual support network for individuals and families. The cost is free, and the patient must be 12 years or older to participate.
Can be accessed at https://www.jdrf.org/t1d-resources/personal-support/.[18]

National Institute of Diabetes and Digestive and Kidney Diseases

This site provides quality education on the different diabetes types including type 1, type 2, gestational diabetes, and monogenic diabetes.
Can be accessed at www.niddk.nih.gov.[19]

Additional Online Resources

- https://diatribe.org: diatribe provides up-to-date diabetes information and tips for people with diabetes. Their mission is to "help individuals better understand their diabetes" and to "make readers happier and healthier."
- diabeteswise.org: helps patients with diabetes technology and to find the right devices for their lifestyle. It is an initiative from Stanford University School of Medicine and people living with diabetes. It is supported by The Leona M. and Harry B. Helmsley Charitable Trust.
- https://diabetessisters.org: helps women with all types of diabetes live healthier, fuller lives by offering education and support services. Managed by women who are living with diabetes.

There are many more Web sites devoted to diabetes education that provide free handouts and other materials for patients and providers. The Internet has been a great source when it comes to availability of information; however, it is important to help patients be selective with the data they access.

The provider must reach out to the local health department. There are free education classes and groups for diabetes support and in some cases, government-funded programs that may help patients of low socioeconomic status.

FINANCIAL RESOURCES

Cost of medications is an important barrier for adherence in patients with diabetes, especially for patients with limited or no health insurance. A study done in New Mexico in a primary care screening program found that patients with newly diagnosed type 2 diabetes (n = 118) failed to seek medical care due to lack of health insurance coverage.[20] In practice, many times we see patients who get lost to follow-up, who then come back in a very deteriorated condition after recovering health insurance coverage.

There are other services aside from medication coverage that are affected by lack of health insurance such as DSMES, podiatry, ophthalmology, dental services, and even obtaining diabetes supplies.

To mitigate these adverse factors, many private and public organizations have come together to assist patients with diabetes.

Patient Assistance Programs

These are private or public programs that offer discounted or free medicines. Qualification for these programs is based on income and age, and it is recommended to have an office staff person designated to handle application processes, medication organization, and proper storage (refrigeration will be needed with insulin products), as for the most part the medications will come to the doctor's office. The patient will need to provide the following additional information:

- Prescription information:
  - Name of each drug
  - Dose
  - Frequency of administration
- Annual gross total household income
- Household size: number of people living together and contributing to the total household income
- State of residence
- Name of insurance if patient is covered.

These are just a selected number of programs that may be found helpful:

- *Medicare Prescription Drug Plan Finder:* if covered under Medicare, patients are eligible for Medicare prescription drug coverage regardless of income, health status, or current prescription coverage.
  - This service provides a personalized list of drug plans that includes costs and other features.
  - For more information, a toll-free number is available: 1-800-MEDICARE (1-800–633–4227)
  - Web site: http://www.medicare.gov/
- *Patient Assistance Connection: by Sanofi*

- o This program offers prescription assistance and vaccines at no cost to qualifying patients.
- o Eligibility criteria:
  - Must be a resident of the United States or the US territories and be under the care of a licensed health care provider authorized to prescribe, dispense, and administer medicine in the United States.
  - Must have no insurance coverage or access to the prescribed product or treatment via insurance.
  - Must have an income at or less than 400% of federal poverty guidelines.
  - If enrolled in Medicare Part D, in addition to the criteria mentioned earlier, must also spend at least 2% of annual household income on prescription medications covered through the Part D plan in the current calendar year.
  - For vaccines, must be 19 years of age or older (except for IMOVAX Rabies and IMOGAM Rabies-HT).
- o To apply: https://www.sanofipatientconnection.com/patient-assistance-connection
- o Or call: 800-633-1610
- *Insulins Valyou Savings: by Sanofi*
  - o This program guarantees the price of insulin prescriptions for 12 consecutive monthly fills. It helps reduce prescription costs but is not for free.
  - o Insulins covered in this program are:
    ADMELOG (insulin lispro injection) 100 Units/mL
    TOUJEO (insulin glargine injection) 300 Units/mL
    LANTUS (insulin glargine injection) 100 Units/mL
    APIDRA (insulin glulisine injection) 100 Units/mL
  - o This offer is not valid for prescriptions submitted for reimbursement to Medicare, Medicaid, VA, DOD, TRICARE, similar federal or state programs, including any state pharmaceutical programs, or commercial/private insurance.
  - o For more information: 833-813-0190
  - o To apply: visit Web site https://www.admelog.com/insulins-valyou-savings-program?utm_source=vanityurl&utm_medium=redirect&utm_campaign=valyou
- *Patient Assistance Program: by Novo Nordisk US*
  - o This program provides diabetes medications at no cost to qualified patients.
  - o Eligibility:
  - o Must be a US citizen or legal resident.
    - Must have an income at or less than 400% of federal poverty guidelines.
    - Must be uninsured or in the Medicare program.
    - Must not be enrolled in or qualify for any other federal, state, or government program such as Medicaid, Low Income Subsidy, or Veterans (VA) Benefits. Exceptions include patients who are Medicaid eligible who have applied for and been denied Medicaid.
    - Available to individuals with job loss due to COVID 19 pandemic.
  - o To apply: visit Web site and download application https://www.novocare.com/diabetes-overview/let-us-help/pap.html or call 866-310-7549
  - o Submit any of these documents for proof of income: 2 most current paycheck stubs, earning statements for all working household members, last year's Federal Income Tax Return (1040), Social Security income, pension, and other income statements, W-2 or 1099 forms, or unemployment benefit statements.

- ○ COVID 19 job loss exception documents: include documentation showing loss of health care benefits (job termination notice, job status change, proof that COBRA benefits are being offered). No proof of income required.
- *Lilly Cares Prescription Assistance: by Eli Lilly and Company*
  - ○ This program helps people obtain diabetes medications if they have no insurance, Medicare Part D, or are underinsured.
  - ○ Eligibility:
    - Income less than ~300% of Federal Poverty Income Level
    - For permanent legal US residents
    - Not enrolled or ineligible for Medicaid or VA benefits.
    - Eligible or enrolled in Medicare Part D Program
    - Patients who have spent $1100.00 or more on medications this calendar year
    - Uninsured patients
  - ○ Diabetes medications must be written for up to 90-day supply
  - ○ Providers use a Lilly care Prescription Form for enrolled patients
  - ○ For more information: call 800-545-6962
  - ○ To apply: https://www.lillycares.com/how-to-apply
  - ○ Diabetes medicines included in the program are:
    Glucagon (glucagon for injection [rDNA origin])
    Humalog U100 (insulin lispro injection)
    Humalog U200 (insulin lispro injection)
    Humalog Mix75/25 (75% insulin lispro protamine suspension, 25% insulin lispro injection [rDNA origin])
    Humalog Mix50/50 (50% insulin lispro protamine suspension, 50% insulin lispro injection [rDNA origin])
    Humulin 70/30 (70% human insulin isophane suspension, 30% human insulin injection [rDNA origin])
    Humulin N (NPH human insulin [rDNA origin] isophane suspension)
    Humulin R (U-100) (regular insulin human injection USP [rDNA origin]) Humulin R (U-500) (regular U-500 [concentrated] insulin human injection USP [rDNA origin])
    Trulicity (dulaglutide) injection
- *Insulin Value Program: by Eli Lilly and Company*
  - ○ Helps patients of all ages regardless of their insurance status: commercial insurance, no insurance, employed, furloughed, or unemployed.
  - ○ Eligibility: because of federal guidelines, seniors in Medicare Part D plans are not eligible for a savings card but can call the Solution Center to see if they are eligible for other options.
  - ○ Provides Lilly insulins for $35.00 per month as a response to COVID 19.
  - ○ To learn more and apply: https://www.insulinaffordability.com/
- *Diabetes Management Supplies: by CR3 Diabetes Association*
  - ○ This program provides reduced-cost diabetes management supplies to uninsured or underinsured individuals who meet household income guidelines.
  - ○ It can provide glucose and testing strips, insulin pumps, and insulin pumps supplies.
  - ○ Application process is through their Web site at https://cr3diabetes.org/application-form/
  - ○ Their contact number is 919-388-7757

- o States covered: WA, WI, WV, FL, WY, NH, NJ, NM, NC, ND, NE, NY, RI, NV, CO, CA, GA, CT, OK, OH, KS, SC, KY, OR, SD, DE, DC, HI, TX, LA, TN, PA, VA, AK, AL, AR, VT, IL, IN, IA, AZ, ID, ME, MD, MA, UT, MO, MN, MI, MT, and MS.
- Savings cards:

Many drugs for diabetes have savings cards. Pharmacists and Web sites are good sources of information for this.

Savings cards allow for a significant reduction in the price of the medication, and some medications can be obtained at very low or $0 copay.

In general medication savings cards are not valid for prescriptions covered by or submitted for reimbursement under Medicare, Medicaid, VA, DOD, or TRICARE, or similar federal or state programs including any state medical pharmaceutical programs.

- o *America's Pharmacy: Prescription discount cards*
  - No enrollment fees, no claim forms, no deductibles, and no questions about health.
  - Patients must search for card or coupon and present them to the pharmacy to get a discount.
  - To apply visit Web site: https://www.americaspharmacy.com/
- o *Choice drug card:*
  - Activated & Ready-To-Use Prescription Discount Card/Coupon. Everyone Can Use This Card—Your Entire Family—*FREE Forever and Reusable!!*
  - Save up to 85% off your prescription medications!
    Population that benefits:
    - People with no health care insurance including students
    - People who have insurance but have high deductibles, noncovered drugs, high copayments, or caps on their benefits.
    - Seniors who fall into the donut-hole of their Medicare Part D
    - Employees who are in their waiting period for health care coverage
    - Employees who cannot afford COBRA payments when they lose their job
    - Employees who cannot afford to cover dependents
    Features and benefits:
    - Save up to 85% off prescription
    - Can be used immediately with no activation required
    - Never expires and reusable
    - Use the card at all your pharmacies
    - Share the card with friends, family, or anyone who needs the savings
    - 100% Free—No Fees EVER
    - No Registration Required
    - Choice drug card never receives your personal information
    - No residency requirements
    - Cheaper than insurance at times, check with your pharmacy
    - Businesses can offer to their employees in place of a prescription plan
- o *Good Rx Prescription Discount Card:*
  - Claims discounts up to 80% on most prescription drugs over 70,000 US pharmacies.
  - Discounts for every member of the family, including pets.
  - No expiration, fees, or obligations.
- *Insulin Syringe Assist: by Becton, Dickinson, and Company*
  - o Provides eligible participants with a 90-day supply of BD syringes via mail.
  - o Eligibility: must decrease to less than Annual Gross Maximum income: $28,000 for single and $38,000 for married households. Also, patient must not have

insulin syringe coverage by any insurer, both private and public (state Medicaid and federal Medicare).
- ○ Copayment to participate is $15.00
- ○ To apply: call 888-367-8517
- ○ Web site: https://www.bd.com/en-us/offerings/capabilities/diabetes-care/insulin-syringes
- ○ Covers residents of all 50 states
- *Walmart $4 Medication List:*
  - ○ This Prescription Program offers select generic oral diabetes medications commonly prescribed at affordable prices: $4.00 for 30-day supply and $10.00 for a 90-day supply. Medications offered are metformin, glimepiride, glipizide, and pioglitazone.
  - ○ Walmart offers the ReliOn brand for Novolin N (NPH vial), Novolin R (regular insulin vial), and Novolin 70/30 (mixed insulin vial) at the price of $25.00 each. In addition, it offers diabetes supplies such as meters and testing strips also at affordable prices.
  - ○ In June 2021 Walmart announced its new analogue insulin ReliOn NovoLog Vials and FlexPens. This insulin is offered at a much lower price: $72.88 per vial and $85.88 per FlexPen box; this saves patients between 58% and 75% off the cash price for branded products.[21]
- *CVS Pharmacy: CVS Health*
  - ○ CVS offers various products and services for patients with diabetes that includes Novo Nordisk's Novolin R, Novolin N, and Novolin 70/30 at $25.00 per vial.
- *Livongo:*
  - ○ Some employers and health plans offer a smart meter, unlimited testing supplies, and expert advice from a Diabetes Educator at no cost to patients.
- *NeedyMeds:* this is a national nonprofit information resource designed to find assistance programs for prescription medications and help with other health care costs. There is a service fee (~ $49.00), and the application process is online. Based on the information provided by the patient, they will determine if he or she qualifies for assistance and will also handle the refill process.
- *Nice Rx:*
  - ○ Provides lower-cost medications for $49.00 per month.
  - ○ Patients apply at https://www.nicerx.com/, are informed of their eligibility status, and are not billed again until their prescription arrives.
  - ○ They also handle the refill process.
- *Rx Outreach:*
  - ○ Rx Outreach is a charitable nonprofit Patient Assistance Program. The program provides access to affordable generic and brand-name medications to qualified individuals and families based on income.
  - ○ To apply call: (800) 769-3880
- *Well Rx:*
  - ○ Offers prescription discounts
  - ○ Locates lowest retail price of medications.
  - ○ Convenience of use of a smartphone app instead of a card.

MOBILE HEALTH APPS FOR DIABETES

Digital health technology, especially digital and health applications ("apps"), has been developing rapidly to help people manage their diabetes. Numerous health-related apps provided on smartphones and other wireless devices are available to support people with diabetes who need to adopt either lifestyle interventions or medication adjustments in response to glucose-monitoring data. However, regulations and guidelines have not caught up with the burgeoning field to standardize how mobile health apps are reviewed and monitored for patient safety and clinical validity.[22]

Mobile health apps may not be a panacea. In 2018 an AHRQ study evaluated 11 randomized controlled trials (clinical vs control) among hundreds of diabetes self-management apps. The results showed that 5 were associated with clinically significant but small improvements in HbA1c. None of the apps demonstrated improvements in quality of life, blood pressure, weight, or BMI. None were high-quality applications to aid in the treatment of diabetes.[22]

Apps are difficult to study. Because apps are never "frozen" in time as a medication; program developers are constantly making improvements. Also, they are never blinded, so placebo effect cannot be ruled out, and typically they are of lower commercial value and have shorter life cycle that does not support the high cost and time involved in conducting randomized controlled trials.[22]

Other issues with mobile apps for the management of diabetes are lack of evidence, inadequate training of health care providers, inaccuracy, lack of clinical validity, variable quality, ease of use, difficulty with interoperability amid other devices, no standardization, does not take into account variability between population of users, data insecurity, and limited privacy protection.

The Food and Drug Administration (FDA) approved mobile apps for insulin titration:

- *WellDoc Blue Star:* insulin titration app that offers more insight into glycemic patterns and advice on diabetes self-management between visits.
- *Voluntis Insulia:* Voluntis enhances treatment experiences by empowering patients and their care team with personalized, algorithm-based digital therapeutics.
- *Sanofi MyDose Coach:* an app designed to help patients with type 2 diabetes titrate basal insulin doses.
- *Glooko:* has a long-acting insulin titration system.
- *Amalgam iSage Rx:* a basal insulin titration system.
- *Hygieia's d-Nav Insulin Guidance Service:* an app that titrates insulin doses for individual patients with type 2 diabetes, regardless of their regimen type and received 510(k) clearance from the FDA.

MENTAL HEALTH AND DIABETES

The ADA recognizes mental health care is an integral part of diabetes management. Because of this, they have developed a Web site devoted to helping patients with diabetes understand the interplay of diabetes and mental health. The Web site offers support and tools for patients and has a link to a Mental Health referral directory.

The Web site is https://www.diabetes.org/healthy-living/mental-health.

CLINICS CARE POINTS

- Diabetes is a very complex chronic condition that requires the individual's engagement and self-management education. Because of this, they need training and should have access to a multidisciplinary team including diabetes educators, dieticians, pharmacists, social workers, prior authorization team members, medication assistance specialists, and mental health providers, in addition to the clinician.

- When dealing with patients resistant to care, it is important to seek understanding of their beliefs and attitudes toward the disease. Helping these patients requires compassion and a true interest in the person so a bridge can be built, and trust between the patient and the provider is established.

- When investigating about resources for patients with diabetes, clinicians must not forget to reach out to their local health department that may already have free programs. In addition, excellent online directories can be found at the ADA Web site, as well as American Heart Association among others.

DISCLOSURES

The author has nothing to disclose.

REFERENCES

1. Centers for Disease Control and Prevention. National diabetes Statistics report. Atlanta, (GA): Centers for Disease Control and Prevention, U.S. Dept of Health and Human Services; 2020. Available at: https://www.cdc.gov/diabetes/data/statistics-report/index.html. July 30th, 2021.
2. Nam S, Chesla C, Stotts NA, et al. Barriers to diabetes management: patient and provider factors. Diabetes Res Clin Pract 2011;93(1):1–9.
3. Tuchman AM. History of diabetes. MD Advis 2013;6(1):8–13.
4. Hirsch IB, Juneja R, Beals JM, et al. The Evolution of Insulin and How it Informs Therapy and Treatment Choices. Endocr Rev 2020;41(5):733–55.
5. Luthra A, Misra A. Escalating cost of oral and injectable antihyperglycemic drugs; are newer medications worth their price? A perspective from India and other developing countries. Diabetes Metab Syndr 2020;14(2):167–9.
6. Cha AE, Cohen RA. Reasons for being uninsured among adults aged 18–64 in the United States, 2019. NCHS Data Brief, no 382. Hyattsville, (MD): National Center for Health Statistics; 2020.
7. Lawton J, Peel E, Parry O, et al. Lay perceptions of type 2 diabetes in Scotland: bringing health services back in. Soc Sci Med 2005;60:1423–35.
8. Anderson RM, Donnelly MB, Dedrick RF. Measuring the attitudes of patients towards diabetes and its treatment. Patient Educ Couns 1990;16:231–45.
9. Farmer A, Kinmonth AL, Sutton S. Measuring beliefs about taking hypoglycemic medication among people with Type 2 diabetes. Diabet Med 2006;23:265–70.
10. de Weerdt I, Visser AP, Kok G, et al. Determinants of active self-care behavior of insulin treated patients with diabetes: implications for diabetes education. Soc Sci Med 1990;30:605–15.
11. Dunn SM. Rethinking the models and modes of diabetes education. Patient Educ Couns 1990;16:281–6.
12. Masaki Y, Okada S, Ota Z. Importance of attitude evaluation in diabetes patient education. Diabetes Res Clin Pract 1990;8:37–44.
13. Centers for Disease Control and Prevention. DSMES _ diabetes self -management and support 2018. https://www.cdc.gov/diabetes/dsmes-toolkit/background/index.html. August 2 2021.
14. Rutledge SA, Masalovich S, Blacher RJ, et al. Diabetes self-management education programs in nonmetropolitan counties — United States, 2016. MMWR Surveill Summ 2017;66(No. SS-10):1–6.
15. Powers MA, Bardsley J, Cypress M, et al. Diabetes Self-Management Education and Support in Type 2 Diabetes: A Joint Position Statement of the American

Diabetes Association, the American Association of Diabetes Educators, and the Academy of Nutrition and Dietetics. J Acad Nutr Diet 2015;115(8):1323–34.

16. American Diabetes Association. Resources. Available at: https://www.diabetes.org/resources. August 2 2021.

17. American Heart Association. Diabetes tools and resources. Available at: https://www.heart.org/en/health-topics/diabetes/diabetes-tools–resources.   August   2 2021.

18. Juvenile Diabetes research Foundation. Get personal support. https://www.jdrf.org/t1d-resources/personal-support/. August 2 2021.

19. National Institute of Diabetes and Digestive and Kidney Diseases. US Department of health and Human Services. National institutes of Health. USA.gov. Available at: https://www.niddk.nih.gov/. August 2 2021.

20. Burge MR, Lucero S, Rassam AG, et al. What are the barriers to medical care for patients with newly diagnosed diabetes mellitus? Diabetes Obes Metab 2000; 2(6):351–4.

21. Walmart revolutionizes insulin access & affordability. 2021. Available at: https://corporate.walmart.com/newsroom/2021/06/29/walmart-revolutionizes-insulin-access-affordability-for-patients-with-diabetes-with-the-launch-of-the-first-and-only-private-brand-analog-insulin. August 2, 2021.

22. Fleming GA, Petrie JR, Bergenstal RM, et al. Diabetes digital app technology: benefits, challenges, and recommendations. a consensus report by the european association for the study of diabetes (EASD) and the American Diabetes Association (ADA) diabetes technology working group. Diabetes Care 2020;43(1): 250–60.

Special Psychosocial Issues in Diabetes Management: Diabetes Distress, Disordered Eating, and Depression

Michael S. Shapiro, PhD

KEYWORDS

- Diabetes distress • Disordered eating • Psychosocial factors in diabetes care

KEY POINTS

- Diabetes care is difficult, made more so by confounding psychosocial issues such as diabetes distress, disordered eating, and mood disorders.
- Screening for these conditions is both critical and feasible for the primary care physician.
- A good understanding of these disorders can inform treatment decisions regarding medication, therapy, and other medical and psychosocial interventions.

INTRODUCTION

Many human maladies are mediated by psychosocial factors, perhaps none more than type 2 diabetes. This is why successful diabetes prevention programs focus on lifestyle factors, including the mitigation of stress, to prevent diabetes onset in people with and without prediabetes.[1,2] This article will focus on 3 special challenges that are often interrelated and mutually self-sustaining (thereby confounding the psychosocial aspects of diabetes management), namely diabetes distress, disordered eating, and clinical depression.

Diabetes Distress

Diabetes is a chronic, relentless disease that, while manageable, requires constant vigilance and effort on the part of the patient. This often results in diabetes distress, which refers to a type of emotional burnout that develops in patients who have had to devote considerable amounts of time and emotional energy to the management of the disease. Signs of diabetes distress include:

- Feelings of frustration and anger in response to the demands of self-care.
- Guilt over the degree to which self-management impacts relationships with friends and family.

Duke/Southern Regional Area Health Education Center, 1601 Owen Drive, Fayetteville, NC 28304, USA
E-mail address: Michael.Shapiro@sr-ahec.org

Prim Care Clin Office Pract 49 (2022) 363–374
https://doi.org/10.1016/j.pop.2021.11.007
0095-4543/22/© 2021 Elsevier Inc. All rights reserved.

- Constant anxiety over food choices, blood sugar levels, and exercise requirements.
- Feelings of defeat and isolation.

It has been estimated that up to 45% of people with diabetes experience diabetes distress.[3] Whereas diabetes distress shares symptoms with major depressive disorder (MDD), 70% of persons with diabetes distress do not meet the criteria for a diagnosis of MDD.[4] As such, diabetes distress may be comorbid with a mood disorder, but it should be viewed as a separate clinical entity that requires attention from the primary care provider, especially because diabetes distress has been shown to impede self-management behaviors.[5]

Assessment of Diabetes Distress

Primary care physicians are well-versed in educating their patients on the medical aspects of diabetes, from cause to prevention to treatment. However, they may neglect warning their patients about the emotional sequelae of diabetes, assuming that these would be self-evident, or relegating such concerns to the scope of a behavioral health provider. Furthermore, the data suggest that providers often find it difficult to distinguish somatic symptoms of depression or diabetes distress from the symptoms of actual physical illness.[6]

Therefore, because diabetes distress may escalate into a major depressive episode, early identification is critical. Screening for diabetes distress can be undertaken with instruments such as the Problem Areas in Diabetes Survey (PAID), which assesses various areas of psychological and emotional distress related to diabetes.[7,8] This 20-question survey elicits patients' opinions regarding the degree to which the disease has impacted their mood, social functioning, and goals for the future. It is easy to administer, easy to interpret, psychometrically sound, and sensitive to change over time (making it useful as a longitudinal tracking instrument).[9,10] Shorter measures (the PAID-1 and PAID-5) have also been developed that are also psychometrically robust and may be more palatable for some patients due to their brevity.[11] The Diabetes Distress Scale is another useful instrument that captures 4 crucial dimensions of distress; emotional burden, regime distress, interpersonal distress, and physician distress.[12] There are multiple forms of this measure (patient, partner, and parents of teen patients), thereby affording a comprehensive view of patient wellbeing.

The Physician Connection

Once diabetes distress has been identified, what can be conducted to help your patient navigate what may become a lifelong or cyclical course of periodic burnout and despair? Multiple studies have shown that diabetes distress contributes to poor glycemic control and compromised self-care, ostensibly due to patients' low self-efficacy, feelings of futility, sense of powerlessness, frustration with the health care system, and exhaustion associated with the day-to-day management of the disease.[13-16] In turn, the primary care provider, who has been working hard to ensure that patient's health and stability, may develop feelings of frustration toward a patient who seems to be undermining the provider's efforts to keep them healthy.

It has been shown that the quality of the patient–physician relationship has a powerful influence on adherence to medication and other self-care directives, with better outcomes noted in patients who have confidence in their health care provider.[17,18] Therefore, supportive, compassionate physicians who understand the interaction between the physical and mental aspects of disease management will be better prepared to sympathize with patients and validate their feelings of frustration and exhaustion.

The Importance of Self-efficacy

Toward the end of supporting a patient emotionally, the data suggest that it is best to target self-efficacy, which is the patient's confidence in their ability to manage their own disease and take responsibility for self-care.[19] Once a patient has been educated on how to accomplish a relatively simple self-care task, such as checking blood sugar, the primary care provider can promote self-efficacy by encouraging short-term goals and praising small victories before introducing the next, more complicated step in self-care, such as being able to inject oneself in a public setting, or when conditions are less than optimal.[20] Once mastery of a small task has been attained and reinforced through the care and encouragement of the provider, the patient's efforts should be praised, and persistence should be lauded. Then, when it is time to learn a more complicated task, or when difficulties arise, self-efficacy can be reinforced by reminding the patient of past successes.[21]

Social and Family Support

In addition to encouraging and fostering self-efficacy, the primary care physician should ensure that patients receive family and social support, which means inviting family and friends to join the patient's lifelong diabetes journey to some degree. Such support has robustly been shown to play a significant role in the successful management of diabetes, and there is a strong direct relationship between perceived social support and a patient's ability to cope with the disease.[22–24] Consequently, the primary care provider should be sure to educate family members on all aspects of treatment, including the importance of practical day-to-day management tasks and adherence to dietary and exercise guidelines. In doing so, the trusted health care provider becomes part of the patient's larger family support system.

Group Support

Outside of the immediate family and the primary health care team, psychosocial support groups can be most effective in mitigating diabetes distress.[25] Whereas individual therapy and group counseling interventions have both been shown to improve quality of life and self-care efficacy in patients with diabetes, group interventions are more cost-effective, and they hold particular appeal for patients who may be tempted to retreat into solitude because they assume that no one can understand their world or truly empathize with the emotional turmoil of diabetes distress.[26] Groups focus on a common goal (learning to cope with diabetes) rather than a common pathology, thereby broadening their appeal. In a group setting venue, the patient sees first-hand that others share their experience. Participants validate each other's feelings while being afforded an opportunity to exchange hints on disease management. In turn, this promotes hopefulness, further fosters self-efficacy, and widens the social support network.

Typically, group interventions directed at chronic disease are of three main types: educational groups (brief, therapist-centered sessions that focus on practical management skills), social/emotional support groups (less structured sessions with a therapist who facilitates free discussions on a number of group-selected topics), and peer-led support groups (in which there is little or no involvement of a mental health or health care professional).[25] Of these, even the groups with the least amount of professional intervention (but lots of mutual education and peer support) have documented efficacy in decreasing anxiety, depression, and diabetes distress while increasing self-management skills and promoting a better quality of life.[27] Primary care providers can refer their patients to regional support groups with the help of the Defeat Diabetes Foundation, which maintains a directory of such groups by state.

DISORDERED EATING

Relative to the general population, patients with diabetes are, by necessity, excessively focused on food, body weight, caloric intake, and eating schedules. It is easy to see how this constant vigilance would predispose a patient to unhealthy eating behaviors, collectively referred to as disordered eating. Disordered eating should be viewed on a spectrum that ranges from specific eating disorders (anorexia nervosa, bulimia nervosa, and binge-eating disorder) to irregular eating patterns that may not warrant a clinical diagnosis in terms of intensity or severity.[28,29] Such behaviors include:

- Severe restriction of food intake,
- Binge eating,
- The use of unhealthy weight-loss strategies, such as self-induced vomiting or skipping meals,
- Preoccupation with food and body image,
- Adaptation of rigid rituals surrounding eating,
- Feelings of shame associated with eating foods that are unwise for a diabetic,
- Manipulation of insulin doses to lose weight (a condition known as diabulimia),
- "Counteracting" bad food choices with excessive exercise.

It has been suggested that up to 40% of patients with diabetes are somewhere on the spectrum between disordered eating and diagnosable eating disorders, of which binge-eating disorder is most common.[30–32] As might be expected, diabetes and disordered eating may influence each other in a cyclical fashion, or one may precede the other. For example, persons with binge-eating disorder may develop insulin resistance and weight gain, which in turn predispose them to diabetes. In patients who already have diabetes, fear of gaining weight or eating the "wrong" foods might predispose them to anorexia nervosa. In any event, disordered eating can significantly increase diabetes mortality and morbidity, and can increase microvascular complications.[29]

Assessment of Disordered Eating

As disordered eating patterns may not always meet the full diagnostic criteria for one of the feeding and eating disorders in the DSM.,[5] and because patients themselves may be unaware that their eating behaviors are not "normal" (depending on things like familiar or cultural perception of "normal" eating behaviors), it is crucial for the primary care provider to screen patients with diabetic regularly for unhealthy eating behaviors. Both the SCOFF (Sick, Control, One, Fat, and Food) and the EDE-Q (Eating Disorder Examination Questionnaire) have been found to be especially useful in the primary care setting.[33] However, such instruments, which are typically used to screen for eating disorders in the general population, may be of limited usefulness for patients with diabetic, as their abnormal eating behaviors may not rise to the clinical threshold of an eating disorder, or their eating behaviors may be "atypical" relative to persons whose eating disorders are unrelated to diabetes.

Moreover, as disordered eating is not a diagnosis in itself (but is, as noted earlier, considered to be on a spectrum of eating disorders), there is no standard definition of this term, no specific diagnostic criteria, and, consequently, no test that is designed specifically to screen for disordered eating in the diabetic population. Instead, it would be useful to use the Eating Disorders Test-26 (EAT-26), which is a validated psychometric measure that identifies risk for eating disorders in the general population.[34] One study on women athletes found that a score of 12 on the EAT-26 serves as a valid cut-score to indicate when someone is at risk for developing disordered eating, which may be a precursor to a fulminant eating disorder.[35] The EAT-26 is a brief self-report measure that is palatable to patients and permits longitudinal monitoring through periodic readministration over time.

Treatment of Disordered Eating

As the gatekeeper of a patient's overall health, the primary care physician becomes the focal point for the treatment of disordered eating. However, a multidisciplinary care team is considered the standard for the treatment of aberrant eating behaviors.[28] In addition to the primary care provider, this team would include a registered dietician, a diabetologist/endocrinologist, and a behavioral health clinician. While the primary care provider oversees medication management, the registered dietician and diabetologist are best equipped to educate the patient and family on dietary and treatment issues; while also monitoring key indicators (such as HbA1c levels). They may also request that the patient keep a food diary, to record not only food intake and eating schedules but also the feelings associated with certain foods, and details about the eating environment that might trigger disordered eating behaviors.[29]

As disordered eating is the result of a convoluted interface between social, psychological, and biological factors, individual therapy is indicated to help the diabetic individual deal with multiple emotional issues. These include grief (over the loss of a "normal" life), acceptance (of having to struggle with a chronic, lifelong illness), body image distortion, recognition, and rejection of maladaptive coping mechanisms, and the delineation of family and environmental factors that contribute to disordered eating. As a prelude to individual therapy, a thorough psychological evaluation would be useful as a way to sort out these issues and establish specific therapeutic goals. A good psychological evaluation will also reveal comorbid diagnoses (such as a mood disorder or anxiety disorder) that might need to be the focus of treatment.[36]

To this end, cognitive behavior therapy (CBT) has the strongest supportive evidence and has been found to be suitable for the treatment of all eating disorders, especially bulimia.[37] As compared with other therapeutic modalities, CBT is time-limited and focuses on providing the patient with skills and techniques to recognize and change the erroneous thoughts that lead to disordered eating. As such, it is more practical than insight-oriented or psychodynamic therapies that focus more on personality, temperament, or past experiences. As previously noted, group therapy allows patients to receive empathy in a safe setting and draw on each other's experiences. Other therapeutic modalities are discussed later in this article.

The Role of Psychopharmacology in Disordered Eating

Until relatively recently, psychopharmacological agents held only a small role in the treatment of eating disorders. Typically, such agents were used to manage some of the psychiatric comorbidities that contribute to eating disorders, such as depression, anxiety, and obsessive-compulsive behaviors. In 1987, during the same year that fluoxetine obtained approval from the US Food and Drug Administration (FDA), an initial study supported its use in the treatment of bulimia.[38] It has since become the preferred medication for this particular eating disorder.[39-41] As then, lisdexamfetamine has been approved (in the United States) for the treatment of binge eating disorder, after studies found it to be effective in reducing the frequency of binge-eating while reducing the obsessive-compulsive component to this disorder.[42,43] Whereas olanzapine has surfaced as a preferred treatment of anorexia nervosa, no other drugs besides fluoxetine and lisdexamfetamine have received FDA approval to date for the treatment of eating disorders.[44,45]

Therefore, while psychotherapeutic interventions should continue to constitute the first line of defense against eating disorders, psychopharmacological treatment of disordered eating can be supported by what is known about how certain medications impact the components of the various systems that are involved in the regulation of appetite and food intake, such as the hypothalamic homeostatic system (ghrelin, leptin, insulin) and the self-regulatory and reward systems of the human brain (serotonin, norepinephrine, glutamate).[46,47] Of course, the choice of a psychopharmacological agent needs to be guided by a number of considerations, such as the exact disordered eating behavior and the presence of any psychiatric comorbidities.

Based on genetic research, it has been suggested that eating disorders should be not only be viewed as psychiatric disorders but also as immune disorders and metabolic disorders as well.[47] As metabolic and immunologic contributions to eating disorders become better understood, novel pharmacologic treatments are sure to follow.

DEPRESSION
The Importance of Depression Screening

As mentioned earlier, individuals with diabetes often experience both depression and diabetes distress, which are distinct but related entities that contribute to poor disease management, as well as a higher risk of mortality. About 45% of adults with diabetes screen positively for both conditions.[48] Furthermore, lifetime rates of depression in patients with type 2 diabetes are between 24% and 29%.[49,50] The symptoms of one can exacerbate the other, and both conditions have been shown to have a negative impact on glycemic control.[48]

Therefore, it is incumbent on the primary care provider to screen their patients with diabetic regularly for both conditions, as recommended by the American Diabetes Association.[51] Screening tools for diabetes distress have already been discussed in this article. Regarding depression, there is an abundance of validated, easy-to-administer screening tools that are sensitive and useful in the primary care setting, such as the Patient Health Questionnaire-9 (PHQ-9) and the Hospital Anxiety and Depression Scale (HADS-D).[52,53] It has been suggested that the HADS-D may be the better of these 2 screening instruments for patients with diabetes.[54]

The results of one meta-analytical study suggest that interventions that focus on attenuating depression and promoting self-efficacy could yield improvements in metabolic control and self-management in patients with diabetic.[55] As such, educating patients on the common comorbidity of depression and diabetes serves as a first step in empowering patients and motivating them to pursue the evaluation and treatment of depressive symptoms. In the context of a collaborative care setting, a comprehensive treatment plan could be constructed to address lifestyle issues that impact depression and diabetes simultaneously, such as exercise and proper nutrition, both of which have been shown to slow disease progression.[56,57] Meta-analyses further suggest that psychotherapeutic interventions, including cognitive-behavior therapy and brief psychodynamic therapy, have contributed to reduced HbA1c levels by a statistically significant degree.[58] This bodes well for patients with diabetic, especially when psychotherapy is combined with traditional psychopharmacological treatments for depression.

Psychopharmacologic Treatment of Depression in Patients with Diabetes

Research suggests that nearly 60% of the total number of patients being treated for depression receive that treatment from a primary care physician.[59] As of 2006, the primary care sector was the largest source of mental health services across all sectors.[60] As such, most primary care physicians have had to become comfortable with the pharmacologic treatment of depression and are well-versed in the use of serotonergic antidepressants (SSRIs, which usually constitute the first line of treatment), atypical antidepressants (eg, bupropion), and tricyclic antidepressants (eg, nortriptyline).

Of these, it has been suggested that the SSRIs may have a synergistic effect on mood and HbA1c levels.[61] Fluoxetine, in particular, has been shown to contribute to improved glycemic control.[62] While nortriptyline has been shown to attenuate depressive symptoms in patients with diabetic, there is evidence that it may actually have an adverse effect on glucose control.[63] The efficacy of bupropion seems to be as effective as the SSRIs in attenuating depression and has also been found to have a favorable impact on weight in patients with diabetic.[64]

Of course, given the intimate connections between mood, food intake, and self-care (including glycemic control), antidepressant medications as a single-modality treatment can be expected to attenuate the symptoms of a mood disorder, but they will not address the complex psychological and social factors that contribute to depression in patients with diabetic. Consequently, treatment is best delivered in the context of an integrated care setting, although more research is needed to delineate exactly how medical, social, and psychological interventions can be integrated optimally for patients with diabetic.[61] For primary care physicians in a single-specialty practice, the following primer on types of counseling, therapy, and behavioral health providers should prove helpful:

Psychotherapeutic and Psychosocial Treatment of Depression in Patients with Diabetes

Psychological and psychosocial interventions have been shown to contribute to a statistically significant reduction in HbA1c levels in patients with diabetic.[58] Although primary care physicians do most of the prescribing when it comes to depression in such patients, they are not behavioral health providers themselves, so they may be less familiar with the psychotherapeutic side of treatment and, in particular, the specific type of mental health professional to whom they should refer their patients.

With the exception of 5 states in the United States in which psychologists can be granted prescription privileges after receiving specialized training, only psychiatrists can prescribe medication. However, there is a virtual alphabet soup of degrees and certifications that apply to nonpsychiatrist mental health clinicians who can help patients with diabetic overcome the primary depression, diabetes distress, and the myriad of social and psychological difficulties that are imposed by their disease. For patients who are served through a clinic that follows integrated care or collaborative care model, access to such clinicians may be relatively simple. For primary care providers who must refer their patients elsewhere for behavioral health services, the following descriptions of behavioral health providers should serve as a guide for both patients and referring physicians:

- Doctoral-level clinical psychologists typically hold a PhD, PsyD (Doctor of Psychology), or EdD (Doctor of Education). In addition to being trained to do therapy, most are also trained in the use of psychological and neuropsychological tests, making them uniquely suited to assist with differential diagnoses when a patient's presentation is confusing, or if there may be multiple psychiatric comorbidities. As such, the information they provide may prove invaluable for treatment planning.
- Master's-level behavioral health providers are usually trained in one or more modalities of psychotherapy or counseling (described later in discussion) and may specialize in the treatment of a particular population or disorder. Their titles vary by state and by training, but may include LPC (Licensed Professional Counselor), Licensed Clinical Social Worker (LCSW), Licensed Marriage and Family Therapist

(LMFT), and Licensed Clinical Mental Health Counselor (LCMHC). These clinicians may be best equipped to provide regular psychosocial support and assist patients with lifestyle changes that may slow disease progression.

Modalities of therapy that are used to treat depression include the following:

- Cognitive behavior therapy (CBT), a short-term, skill-based intervention that focuses on recognizing and changing "negative" or erroneous thoughts that contribute to depressed mood and, for patients with disordered eating, distorted body image.
- Supportive Psychotherapy, which emphasizes the therapeutic alliance between clinician and patient, to the end of alleviating symptoms and maintaining, restoring, or improving self-esteem.
- Brief Psychodynamic Therapy, which unearths and examines troubling feelings or thoughts that interfere with occupational and social functioning.
- Interpersonal Therapy, which is a highly structured, time-limited form of psychotherapy that centers on resolving interpersonal problems and the attenuation of symptoms.
- Acceptance and commitment therapy (ACT), which helps patients learn how to face and accept their feelings rather than avoiding, denying, or struggling with them; to the end of responding to those feelings appropriately.

Of these therapeutic modalities, CBT has the strongest empirical support in the treatment of depression.[65] However, before referring a patient for psychotherapy, primary care physicians should first think about the goal they are trying to achieve: alleviation of depressive symptoms or improved glycemic control. While a number of studies validate the use of psychotherapy for the attenuation of depression, further investigation has been called for to determine whether or not these psychosocial interventions result in better physical health outcomes.[66] In any event, when it comes to the diabetic patient with depression, any psychosocial intervention should always include a focus on issues that might not apply to the nondiabetic depressed patient, such as adherence to diabetic treatment regimens as well physical and nutritional recommendations.[61] Once again, this comprehensive approach to the biological, psychological, and social aspects of diabetes might best be affected in an integrated-care setting.

SUMMARY

Type 2 diabetes can be quite vexing to the primary care physician because its successful management entails so many factors over which the physician has no control, particularly the patient's willingness to adhere to medical treatment as well as dietary restrictions, exercise recommendations, and other aspects of self-care. The physician's job becomes even more complicated when diabetes is compounded by diabetes distress, disordered eating, and clinical depression. Fortunately, there are evidence-based pharmacologic and psychosocial approaches to each of these confounding conditions. The astute primary care physician who is attuned to each of these conditions and their prospective interventions is in the best position to affect positive outcomes, especially when working as part of a treatment team that includes psychotherapists, registered dieticians, diabetologists, and exercise counselors.

CLINICS CARE POINTS

- Diabetes distress, disordered eating, and depression are common psychosocial conditions that confound the treatment of diabetes.

- Diabetes distress and disordered eating may go unrecognized and untreated because they do not meet the clinical criteria of a diagnosable mood disorder or eating disorder, respectively.

- There are practical, validated screening measures for these disorders. These screening measures should become part of the primary care physician's arsenal of diagnostic tools.

- It is most helpful for the primary care physician to empower the patient by promoting self-efficacy and encouraging family support.

- Psychopharmacology has a role in treating these conditions: SSRIs may have a synergistic effect on mood and HbA1c levels, and bupropion has been found to have a favorable impact on weight in patients with diabetic.

- Behavioral health interventions have been shown to contribute to HbA1c reduction in patients with diabetic.

DISCLOSURE

The author has nothing to disclose.

REFERENCES

1. Knowler WC, Barrett-Connor E, Fowler SE, et al. Reduction in the incidence of type 2 diabetes with lifestyle intervention or metformin. N Engl J Med 2002;346(6):393–403.
2. Li G, Zhang P, Wang J, et al. The long-term effect of lifestyle interventions to prevent diabetes in the China Da Qing Diabetes Prevention Study: a 20-year follow-up study. Lancet 2008;371(9626):1783–9.
3. Fisher L, Hessler DM, Polonsky WH, et al. When is diabetes distress clinically meaningful?: establishing cut points for the Diabetes Distress Scale. Diabetes Care 2012;35(2):259–64.
4. Fisher L, Mullan JT, Arean P, et al. Diabetes distress but not clinical depression or depressive symptoms is associated with glycemic control in both cross-sectional and longitudinal analyses. Diabetes Care 2010;33(1):23–8.
5. Fisher L, Glasgow RE, Strycker LA. The relationship between diabetes distress and clinical depression with glycemic control among patients with type 2 diabetes. Diabetes Care 2010;33(5):1034–6.
6. Barley EA, Murray J, Walters P, et al. Managing depression in primary care: A meta-synthesis of qualitative and quantitative research from the UK to identify barriers and facilitators. BMC Fam Pract 2011;12:47.
7. Kreider KE. Diabetes distress or major depressive disorder? A practical approach to diagnosing and treating psychological comorbidities of diabetes. Diabetes Ther 2017;8(1):1–7.
8. Polonsky WH, Anderson BJ, Lohrer PA, et al. Assessment of diabetes-related distress. Diabetes Care 1995;18(6):754–60.
9. Welch GW, Jacobson AM, Polonsky WH. The problem areas in diabetes scale. An evaluation of its clinical utility. Diabetes Care 1997;20(5):760–6.
10. Welch G, Weinger K, Anderson B, et al. Responsiveness of the Problem Areas In Diabetes (PAID) questionnaire. Diabet Med 2003;20(1):69–72.
11. McGuire BE, Morrison TG, Hermanns N, et al. Short-form measures of diabetes-related emotional distress: the Problem Areas in Diabetes Scale (PAID)-5 and PAID-1. Diabetologia 2010;53(1):66–9.
12. Polonsky WH, Fisher L, Earles J, et al. Assessing psychosocial distress in diabetes: development of the diabetes distress scale. Diabetes Care 2005;28(3):626–31.

13. Delahanty LM, Grant RW, Wittenberg E, et al. Association of diabetes-related emotional distress with diabetes treatment in primary care patients with Type 2 diabetes. Diabet Med 2007;24(1):48–54.
14. Fisher L, Hessler D, Glasgow RE, et al. REDEEM: a pragmatic trial to reduce diabetes distress. Diabetes Care 2013;36(9):2551–8.
15. Hessler D, Fisher L, Glasgow RE, et al. Reductions in regimen distress are associated with improved management and glycemic control over time. Diabetes Care 2014;37(3):617–24.
16. King DK, Glasgow RE, Toobert DJ, et al. Self-efficacy, problem solving, and social-environmental support are associated with diabetes self-management behaviors. Diabetes Care 2010;33(4):751–3.
17. Rosland AM, Heisler M, Piette JD. The impact of family behaviors and communication patterns on chronic illness outcomes: a systematic review. J Behav Med 2012;35(2):221–39.
18. Golin CE, DiMatteo MR, Leake B, et al. A diabetes-specific measure of patient desire to participate in medical decision making. Diabetes Educ 2001;27(6):875–86.
19. Krichbaum K, Aarestad V, Buethe M. Exploring the connection between self-efficacy and effective diabetes self-management. Diabetes Educ 2003;29(4):653–62.
20. Morrison G, Weston P. Self-efficacy: a tool for people with type 1 diabetes managed by continuous subcutaneous insulin infusion. J Diabetes Nurs 2013;17:32–7.
21. Margolis H, McCabe P. Self-efficacy: A key to improving the motivation of struggling learners. Clearing House 2004;77:241–9.
22. Tol A, Baghbanian A, Rahimi A, et al. The relationship between perceived social support from family and diabetes control among patients with diabetes type 1 and type 2. J Diabetes Metab Disord 2011;10:1–8.
23. Rintala TM, Jaatinen P, Paavilainen E, et al. Interrelation between adult persons with diabetes and their family: a systematic review of the literature. J Fam Nurs 2013;19(1):3–28.
24. Ramkisson S, Pillay BJ, Sibanda W. Social support and coping in adults with type 2 diabetes. Afr J Prim Health Care Fam Med 2017;9(1):e1–8.
25. van der Ven N. Psychosocial group interventions in diabetes care. Diabetes Spectr 2003;16(2):88–95.
26. Imazu MF, Faria BN, de Arruda GO, et al. Effectiveness of individual and group interventions for people with type 2 diabetes. Rev Lat Am Enfermagem 2015;23(2):200–7.
27. Liu Y, Han Y, Shi J, et al. Effect of peer education on self-management and psychological status in type 2 diabetes patients with emotional disorders. J Diabetes Investig 2015;6(4):479–86.
28. Larrañaga A, Docet MF, García-Mayor RV. Disordered eating behaviors in type 1 diabetic patients. World J Diabetes 2011;2(11):189–95.
29. Pereira RF, Alvarenga M. Disordered eating: identifying, treating, preventing, and differentiating it from eating disorders. Diabetes Spectr 2007;20(3):141–8.
30. García-Mayor RV, García-Soidán FJ. Eating disorders in type 2 diabetic people: brief review. Diabetes Metab Syndr 2017;11:221–4.
31. Papelbaum M, Appolinário JC, Moreira Rde O, et al. Prevalence of eating disorders and psychiatric comorbidity in a clinical sample of type 2 diabetes mellitus patients. Braz J Psychiatry 2005;27(2):135–8.

32. Raevuori A, Suokas J, Haukka J, et al. Highly increased risk of type 2 diabetes in patients with binge eating disorder and bulimia nervosa. Int J Eat Disord 2015; 48(6):555–62.

33. Seferovic A, Dianes GN, Juan B, et al. What is the best screening tool for eating disorders in the primary care setting? Evidence-Based Practice 2019;22(3):12.

34. Garner DM, Garfinkel PE. The eating attitudes test: an index of the symptoms of anorexia nervosa. Psychol Med 1979;9(2):273–9.

35. Haase AM. Weight perception in female athletes: associations with disordered eating correlates and behavior. Eat Behav 2011;12:64–7.

36. Anderson DA, Donahue J, Ehrlich LE, Gorrell S. Psychological assessment of the eating disorders. The Oxford handbook of eating disorders. 2018; 211–221.

37. Murphy R, Straebler S, Cooper Z, et al. Cognitive behavioral therapy for eating disorders. Psychiatr Clin North Am 2010;33(3):611–27.

38. Freeman CP, Hampson M. Fluoxetine as a treatment for bulimia nervosa. Int J Obes 1987;11(Suppl 3):171–7.

39. Aigner M, Treasure J, Kaye W, et al. World Federation of Societies of Biological Psychiatry (WFSBP) guidelines for the pharmacological treatment of eating disorders. World J Biol Psychiatry 2011;12:400–43.

40. Fluoxetine in the treatment of bulimia nervosa. A multicenter, placebo-controlled, double-blind trial. Fluoxetine Bulimia Nervosa Collaborative Study Group. Arch Gen Psychiatry 1992;49(2):139–47.

41. Kaye WH, Weltzin TE, Hsu LK, et al. An open trial of fluoxetine in patients with anorexia nervosa. J Clin Psychiatry 1991;52:464.

42. McElroy SL, Hudson J, Ferreira-Cornwell MC, et al. Lisdexamfetamine dimesylate for adults with moderate to severe binge eating disorder: results of two pivotal phase 3 randomized controlled trials. Neuropsychopharmacology 2016;41: 1251–60.

43. McElroy SL, Hudson JI, Mitchell JE, et al. Efficacy and safety of lisdexamfetamine for treatment of adults with moderate to severe binge eating disorder: a randomized clinical trial. JAMA Psychiatry 2015;72:235–46.

44. Andries A, Frystyk J, Flyvbjerg A, et al. Dronabinol in severe, enduring anorexia nervosa: a randomized controlled trial. Int J Eat Disord 2014;47:18.

45. Frank GK, Shott ME, Hagman JO. The partial dopamine D2 receptor agonist aripiprazole is associated with weight gain in adolescent anorexia nervosa. Int J Eat Disord 2017;5:447.

46. Practice guideline for eating disorders. American Psychiatric Association. Am J Psychiatry 1993;150(2):212–28.

47. Himmerich H, Treasure J. Psychopharmacological advances in eating disorders. Expert Rev Clin Pharmacol 2018;11(1):95–108.

48. Snoek J, Bremmer MA, Hermanns N. Constructs of depression and distress in diabetes: time for an appraisal. Lancet Diabetes Endocrinol 2015;3:450–60.

49. Eiber R, Berlin I, Grimaldi A, et al. Insulin-dependent diabetes and psychiatric pathology: general clinical and epidemiologic review. Encephale 1997;23:351–7.

50. Geffken GR, Ward HE, Staab JP, et al. Psychiatric morbidity in endocrine disorders. Psychiatr Clin North Am 1998;21:473–89.

51. American Diabetes Association. 4. Lifestyle Management. Diabetes Care 2017; 40(Suppl 1):S33–43.

52. Kroenke K, Spitzer RL, Williams JB. The PHQ-9: validity of a brief depression severity measure. J Gen Intern Med 2001;16(9):606–13.

53. Zigmond AS, Snaith RP. The hospital anxiety and depression scale. Acta Psychiatr Scand 1983;67:361–70.

54. Reddy P, Philpot B, Ford D, et al. Identification of depression in diabetes: the efficacy of PHQ-9 and HADS-D. Br J Gen Pract 2010;60(575):e239–45.
55. Brown SA, Garcia AA, Brown A, et al. Biobehavioral determinants of glycemic control in type 2 diabetes: a systematic review and meta-analysis. Patient Educ Couns 2016;99(10):1558–67.
56. Glasgow RE, Boles SM, McKay G, et al. The D-Net diabetes self-management program: long-term implementation, outcomes, and generalization results. Prev Med 2003;36:410–9.
57. Newman S, Steed L, Mulligan K. Self-management interventions for chronic illness. Lancet 2004;364:1523–37.
58. Ismail K, Winkley K, Rabe-Hesketh S. Systematic review and meta-analysis of randomised controlled trials of psychological interventions to improve glycaemic control in patients with type 2 diabetes. Lancet 2004;363(9421):1589–97.
59. Frank RG, Huskamp HA, Pincus HA. Aligning incentives in the treatment of depression in primary care with evidence-based practice. Psychiatr Serv 2003;54(5):682–7.
60. Wang PS, Demler O, Olfson M, et al. Changing profiles of service sectors used for mental health care in the United States. Am J Psychiatry 2006;163(7):1187–98.
61. Markowitz SM, Gonzalez JS, Wilkinson JL, et al. A review of treating depression in diabetes: emerging findings. Psychosomatics 2011;52(1):1–18.
62. Goodnick PJ. Use of antidepressants in treatment of comorbid diabetes mellitus and depression as well as in diabetic neuropathy. Ann Clin Psychiatry 2001;13:31–4.
63. Lustman PJ, Griffith LS, Clouse RE, et al. Effects of nortriptyline on depression and glycemic control in diabetes: results of a double-blind, placebo-controlled trial. Psychosom Med 1997;59:241–50.
64. Jain AK, Kaplan RA, Gadde KM, et al. Bupropion SR vs. placebo for weight loss in obese patients with depressive symptoms. Obes Res 2002;10:1049–56.
65. Cuijpers P, van Straten A, Andersson G, et al. Psychotherapy for depression in adults: a meta-anaysis of comparative outcome studies. J Consult Clin Psychol 2008;76:909–22.
66. Steed L, Cooke D, Newman S. A systematic review of psychosocial outcomes following education, self-management and psychological interventions in diabetes mellitus. Patient Educ Couns 2003;51(1):5–15.

Printed and bound by CPI Group (UK) Ltd, Croydon, CR0 4YY

03/10/2024

01040405-0016